CONTENTS

KU-415-182

Introduction

Food and Nutrition is the eighty-eighth volume in the **Issues** series. The aim of this series is to offer up-to-date information about important issues in our world.

Food and Nutrition looks at healthy eating and food safety.

The information comes from a wide variety of sources and includes:
Government reports and statistics
Newspaper reports and features
Magazine articles and surveys
Website material
Literature from lobby groups
and charitable organisations.

It is hoped that, as you read about the many aspects of the issues explored in this book, you will critically evaluate the information presented. It is important that you decide whether you are being presented with facts or opinions. Does the writer give a biased or an unbiased report? If an opinion is being expressed, do you agree with the writer?

Food and Nutrition offers a useful starting-point for those who need convenient access to information about the many issues involved. However, it is only a starting-point. At the back of the book is a list of organisations which you may want to contact for further information.

*****

Food and Nutrition

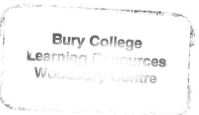

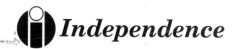

Independence

Educational Publishers
Cambridge

First published by Independence
PO Box 295
Cambridge CB1 3XP
England

British Library Cataloguing in Publication Data
Food and Nutrition – (Issues Series)
I. Donnellan, Craig II. Series
613.2

ISBN 1 86168 289 1

Printed in Great Britain
MWL Print Group Ltd

Typeset by
Claire Boyd

Cover
The illustration on the front cover is by
Pumpkin House.

Adult nutrition

The basics. Information from EUFIC

Introduction

Every day we are bombarded with nutrition and health messages and a seemingly endless array of concerns about lifestyle and diet. Healthy eating and a healthful way of life are important to how we look, feel and how much we enjoy life. The right lifestyle decisions, with a routine of good food and regular exercise, can help us make the most of what life has to offer. Making smart food choices early in life and through adulthood can also help reduce the risk of certain conditions such as obesity, heart disease, hypertension, diabetes, certain cancers and osteoporosis.

Key factors of a healthy diet

Enjoy the wide variety of foods

This concept is the most consistent health message in dietary recommendations around the world. We need more than 40 different nutrients for good health and no single food can supply them all. That's why consumption of a wide variety of foods (including fruits, vegetables, cereals and grains, meats, fish and poultry, dairy products and fats and oils) is necessary for good health and any food can be enjoyed as part of a healthy diet.

Some studies have linked dietary variety with longevity. In any event, choosing a variety of foods adds to the enjoyment of meals and snacks.

Eat regularly

Eating is one of life's great pleasures and it's important to take time to stop, relax and enjoy mealtimes and snacks. Scheduling eating times also ensures that meals are not missed, resulting in missed nutrients that are often not compensated for by subsequent meals. This is especially important for school children, adolescents and the elderly.

EUFIC

Breakfast is particularly important as it helps kick-start the body by supplying energy after the all-night fast. Breakfast also appears to help control weight. All mealtimes offer the opportunity for social and family interaction. So whether it is three square meals or six mini-meals or snacks, the aim is to make healthy choices you can enjoy.

Balance and moderation

Balancing your food intake means getting enough, but not too much, of each type of nutrient. If portion sizes are kept reasonable, there is no need to eliminate favourite foods. There are no 'good' or 'bad' foods, only good or bad diets. Any food can fit into a healthy lifestyle by remembering moderation and balance.

Moderate amounts of all foods can help ensure that energy (calories) intake is controlled and that excessive amounts of any one food or food component are not eaten. If you choose a high fat snack, choose a lower fat option at the next meal. Examples of reasonable serving sizes are 75-100 grams (the size of a palm) of meat, one medium piece of fruit, 1/2 cup raw pasta or one scoop of ice cream (50g). Ready-prepared meals offer a handy means of portion control and they often have the energy (calorie) value listed on the pack.

Maintain a healthy body weight and feel good

A healthy weight varies between individuals and depends on many factors including gender, height, age and hereditary.

Excess body fat results when more calories are eaten than are needed. Those extra calories can come from any source – protein, fat, carbohydrate or alcohol – but fat is the most concentrated source of calories.

Physical activity is a good way of increasing the energy (calories) expended and it can also lead to feelings of well-being. The message is simple: if you are gaining weight eat less and be more active.

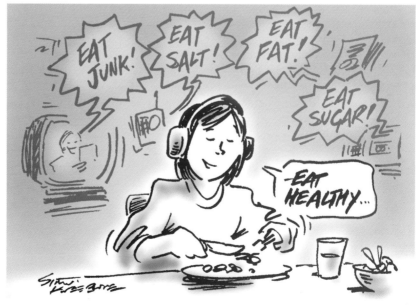

Don't forget your fruits and vegetables

Many Europeans do not meet the recommendations for at least five servings of fruits and vegetables daily. Numerous studies have shown an association between the intake of these foods and a decreased risk of cardiovascular disease and certain cancers. An increased intake of fruits and vegetables has also been associated with decreased blood pressure. People can fill up on fresh fruit and vegetables because they are good sources of nutrients and the majority are naturally low in fat and calories.

Nutritionists are paying much more attention to fruits and vegetables as 'packages' of nutrients and other constituents that are healthful for humans. The 'antioxidant hypothesis' has drawn attention to the role of micronutrients found in fruits and vegetables like vitamins C and E, as well as a number of other natural protective substances. The carotenes (beta-carotene, lutein and lycopene), the flavonoids (phenolic compounds that are widespread in commonly consumed fruits and vegetables such as apples and onions and beverages derived from plants like tea, cocoa and red wine) and the phytoestrogens (principally iso-flavones and lignans) are being demonstrated to have beneficial roles in human health.

Base the diet on foods rich in carbohydrates

Most dietary guidelines recommend a daily diet in which at least 55 of the total calories come from carbo-hydrates. This means making more than half of our daily food intake consist of carbohydrate-containing foods such as grains, pulses, beans, fruits, vegetables and sugars. Choosing wholegrain bread, pasta and other cereals will help to boost fibre intake.

Although the body treats all carbohydrates in the same way regardless of their source, carbo-hydrates are often split into 'complex' and 'simple' carbohydrates. Complex carbohydrates that come from plants are called starch and fibres, and these are found for example in cereal grains, vegetables, breads, seeds, legumes

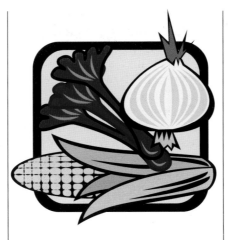

and beans. These carbohydrates consist of long strands of many simple carbohydrates linked together.

Simple carbohydrates (some-times called simple sugars) are found for example in table sugar, fruits, sweets, jams, soft drinks, fruit juices, honey, jellies and syrups. Both complex and simple carbohydrates provide the same amount of energy (4 calories per gram) and both can contribute to tooth decay, especially when oral hygiene is poor.

Drink plenty of fluids

Adults need to drink at least 1.5 litres of fluid daily, even more if it's hot or they are physically active. Plain water is a good source of liquid but variety can be both pleasant and healthy. Choose alternative fluids from juices, soft drinks, tea, coffee and milk.

Fats in moderation

Fat is a nutrient in food that is essential for good health. Fats provide a ready source of energy and enable the body to absorb, circulate and store the fat-soluble vitamins A, D, E and K. Fat-containing foods are needed to supply 'essential fatty acids' that the body cannot make. For example, oil-rich fish and fish oil supplements are rich sources of the omega-3 polyunsaturated fatty acids (n-3 PUFAs) alpha linolenic acid (LNA), eicosapentaenoic acid (EPA) and docosahexaenoic acid (DHA). These, along with omega-6 polyunsaturated fatty acids (n-6 PUFAs) such as linoleic acid and arachidonic acid (AA), must be consumed in the diet.

Too much fat however, especially saturated fats, can lead to adverse health effects such as overweight and high cholesterol and increase the risk of heart disease and some cancers.

Limiting the amount of fat, especially saturated fat in the diet – but not cutting it out entirely – is the best advice for a healthy diet. Most dietary recommendations are that less than 30% of the day's total calories should come from fat and less than 10% of the day's total calories should come from saturated fat.

Balance the salt intake

Salt (NaCl) is made up of sodium and chloride. Sodium is a nutrient and is present naturally in many foods. Sodium and chloride are important in helping the body to maintain fluid balance and to regulate blood pressure.

For most people, any excess sodium passes straight through the body, however, in some people it can increase blood pressure. Reducing the amount of salt in the diet of those who are sensitive to salt may reduce the risk of high blood pressure. The relationship between salt intake and blood pressure is still unclear and individuals should consult their doctor for advice.

Start now – and make changes gradually

Making changes gradually, such as eating one more fruit/portion of vegetables each day, cutting back on portion sizes, or taking the stairs instead of the lift, means that the changes are easier to maintain.

Why is physical activity also important?

The advise for increased physical activity is strongly linked to overall healthy lifestyle recommendations because it affects energy balance and the risk of lifestyle-related diseases. Over the past few years, many position papers have set out the importance of moderate physical activity for good health. These reports indicate that being physically active for at least 30 minutes daily reduces the risk of developing obesity, heart disease, diabetes, hypertension and colon cancer, all of which are major contributors to morbidity and mortality in Europe. In addition, in both children and adults, physical activity is related to improvements in body flexibility, aerobic endurance, agility and coordination, strengthening of bones and muscles, lower body fat levels, blood fats, blood pressure and reduced risk of hip fractures in women. Physical activity makes you feel better physically and encourages a more positive mental outlook.

Increases in physical activity levels are needed in every age group and recommendations are that adults be physically active for at least 30 minutes on most days of the week.

The responsibility for promoting healthy diets and increasing levels of physical activity must involve the active participation of many groups including governments, health professionals, the food industry, the media and consumers. There is a shared responsibility to help promote healthy diets that are low in fat, high in complex carbohydrates and that contain large amounts of fresh fruits and vegetables, along with regular amounts of physical activity.

Ultimately, it is consumers who choose which foods to eat and their choices are influenced by a large number of factors such as quality, price, taste, custom, availability, and convenience. Consumer education, the development and implementation of food-based dietary guidelines, nutrition labelling, nutrition education in schools and increased opportunities for physical activity can all help to improve the nutritional well-being of people.

■ The above information is from EUFIC's website which can be found at www.eufic.org

© 2004, EUFIC

UK child obesity crisis

Information from the International Obesity TaskForce

Obesity and overweight rates have risen dramatically among English schoolchildren in the past five years and are four times higher than 30 years ago, according to a new report from the International Obesity TaskForce released today (12 May 2004).

The latest figures, based on official data from the Health Survey for England for 2001/2, show that more than one in four children are overweight and 6-7% are classified as obese. Applied throughout the UK, it would mean around 2.4 million children are affected by overweight, including 700,000 who are obese.

An analysis of trends reveals that rates of overweight among both boys and girls in the 7-11 year age group are four times the level found 30 years ago. The original overweight figure in 1974 was 7%, rose to 20% in 1998, and leapt even higher to 27% four years later. The narrower band of obese children in this age group increased from 1% in 1974 to 7% in 2001/2.

The estimates use IOTF definitions which provide strict conservative estimates which align childhood rates with the official WHO classification for adult overweight and obesity. The figures are calculated using a different method

to the Department of Health's centiles standard which has indicated childhood obesity has risen threefold over 10 years.

The new figures for England were released alongside a new report on childhood obesity worldwide, which warned that 155 million school-age children were now overweight or obese. One in four children in England are overweight compared with one in 10 worldwide.

Dr Tim Lobstein, co-ordinator of the IOTF's childhood obesity group, said the latest figures for England show that the driving force

behind the obesity epidemic is getting stronger. 'Urgent government action is needed. It isn't enough to expect individuals and parents to cope with this on their own. The environmental factors such as the targeted marketing of children as consumers of high fat, sugar and salty foods needs to be tackled urgently,' he added.

■ The above information is from an IOTF Press Release. For further information visit their website which can be found at www.iotf.org

© International Obesity TaskForce

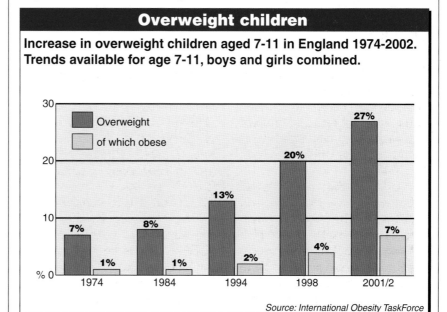

Overweight children

Increase in overweight children aged 7-11 in England 1974-2002. Trends available for age 7-11, boys and girls combined.

Source: International Obesity TaskForce

Teenagers 'too idle' to bother with good food

By Robert Uhlig,
Food Correspondent

Teenagers know which foods are good for them but cannot be bothered to eat healthily or learn to cook properly, a study has shown.

Although three-quarters associate a good diet with long-term health, few can make more than toast and most choose crisps and chocolates rather than fruit.

Among those who do eat fruit, laziness puts them off anything that requires peeling.

'If we buy grapes I eat loads and loads,' a 17-year-old middle-class boy said. 'I just pick them out of the fridge. Oranges you have to peel and that is a chore.'

Four out of 10 teenagers surveyed for the Institute of Grocery Distribution did not eat breakfast. Almost half ate at a fast food restaurant at least once a week, more out of idleness and a desire for convenience than for any other reason.

'I have crisps for breakfast so I can have them on the bus,' a 15-year-old girl said.

When they arrive at school, few teenagers eat healthily. More than half eat junk food or buy fatty snacks and fizzy drinks from the shops rather than eat a school dinner or a packed lunch.

Only one in six buys fruit, vegetables or yogurts.

'In the morning I have cereal,' a 17-year-old boy said. 'But sometimes I can't be bothered so I just have a drink. At break time at school I might have three chocolate bars or a burger. Today I had a burger.'

Diets worsen at weekends and during holidays. A 16-year-old girl was typical of the two in five teenagers who miss breakfast because they stay in bed.

She said: 'At weekends or in the holidays I don't usually eat until the evening because I sleep more during the day.'

Few teenagers associate eating with regular meal times and most lack the skill to prepare anything more than a ready meal. While six out of 10 of those asked knew how to use a microwave, less than a quarter had ever made a pasta sauce.

The study, which said the number of obese people had almost tripled since the present generation of teenagers was born, will make worrying reading for the Government. It is facing an obesity epidemic that is expected to have profound implications for the future health of the nation.

Few teenagers associate eating with regular meal times and most lack the skill to prepare anything more than a ready meal

'Instant gratification is at the forefront of teenagers' demands,' the survey says. 'Issues such as health and nutrition rarely register in the teenage mind and matter only later in life.'

A 17-year-old boy said: 'I will eat junk food until I am 30 then start acting like a grown-up.'

■ Less than half of family doctor organisations have services for overweight patients despite the growth in obesity and nationally approved guidelines for them to follow.

A survey by the health analysts, Dr Foster, found that more than half of primary care organisations had failed to establish weight management clinics.

A third of GPs had no direct access to dietitians, half of primary care organisations had no strategies to audit GPs' work with fat patients and some areas refused to provide money for GPs to prescribe anti-obesity drugs.

Obesity is said to cost the country more than £2 billion a year, with £500 million being spent directly by the NHS.

The National Institute of Clinical Excellence has recommended that GPs tackle patients' obesity first by urging a change in diet, recommending exercise then prescribing drugs.

Very obese patients should finally be referred to hospital with a view to surgery, the institute says.

A quarter of women and one in five men are obese, compared with eight per cent and six per cent in 1980.

Consumption of fruit and vegetables

The proportion eating the recommended amount increases with age. No young men (aged 19-24) interviewed had consumed five or more portions a day and only 4 per cent of young women had done so.

Average daily consumption of five or more portions of fruit and vegetables, 2000-01. Great Britain

Source: National Diet Nutrition Survey, Office for National Statistics

Healthy eating

A whole diet approach

The importance of a healthy and varied diet

A good diet is important for good heath. A healthy and varied diet can help to maintain a healthy body weight, enhance general wellbeing and reduce the risk of a number of diseases including heart disease, stroke, cancer, diabetes and osteoporosis.

What is a healthy diet?

A healthy diet is a diet based on breads, potatoes and other cereals and is rich in fruit and vegetables. A healthy diet will include moderate amounts of milk and dairy products, meat, fish or meat/milk alternatives, and limited amounts of foods containing fat or sugar.

No single food can provide all the essential nutrients that the body needs. Therefore it is important to consume a wide variety of foods to provide adequate intakes of vitamins, minerals and dietary fibre, which are important for health. This article explains how to achieve a healthy diet.

The Balance of Good Health, putting advice into practice

The Government's *Balance of Good Health* is a model of how to eat healthily and is based on the 8 guidelines for a healthy diet (see below). It shows the types and proportions of different foods that should be eaten over a period of time. The *Balance of Good Health* applies to all healthy individuals over five years of age, and can be gradually applied for pre-school children, but does not apply to individuals with special dietary requirements. If you are under medical supervision you should check with your doctor to see whether you should use this guide.

You should choose a variety of foods from each of these four food groups every day:
- bread, other cereals and potatoes
- fruit and vegetables
- milk and dairy foods
- meat, fish and alternatives

**BRITISH
Nutrition
FOUNDATION**

Foods in the fifth group, i.e. foods containing fat and foods containing sugar, can be eaten sparingly as part of a healthy balanced diet but should not be eaten instead of foods from the other food groups, or too often or in large amounts. Having a variety of foods in the diet is important for health – it is not necessary to follow the model at every meal, but rather over a day or two.

8 guidelines for a healthy diet
- Enjoy your food
- Eat a variety of different foods
- Eat the right amount to be a healthy weight
- Eat plenty of foods rich in starch and fibre
- Eat plenty of fruit and vegetables
- Don't eat too many foods that contain a lot of fat
- Don't have sugary foods and drinks too often
- If you drink alcohol, drink sensibly

Fruit and vegetables
What counts?
Fresh, frozen, dried and canned fruit and vegetables all count. Also, 100% fruit or vegetable juice and pure fruit juice smoothies count. Beans and pulses, such as baked beans and lentils also contribute to this group.

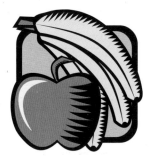

How much should you eat?
Most of us should eat more!

Choose a wide variety and aim to eat at least 5 different portions a day. A portion is approximately 80g (e.g. 1 medium apple, a cereal bowl of salad or 3 heaped tablespoons of peas). Servings of fruit juice, vegetable juice or smoothies can only count as one portion per day no matter how much you drink. Beans and pulses (i.e. haricot, kidney, baked, soya and butter beans, chickpeas and lentils) only count once per day no matter how many different types you eat.

Look out for the Government's 5 A Day logo on pre-packed fruit and vegetables; some food manufacturers have their own logos.

Why eat these foods?
These foods provide:
Vitamin C: needed for healthy skin and tissue, also to aid the absorption of iron
Carotenes: required for growth and development
Folate:* needed for red blood cells
Fibre: keeps the gut healthy and helps prevent constipation
Carbohydrate: a source of energy
Phytochemicals: may help protect against some diseases

Healthy eating tips
- Choose fruit or chopped vegetables as a snack
- Add dried or fresh fruit to breakfast cereals
- Have a salad with sandwiches or with pizza
- Add vegetables to casseroles and stews and fruit to desserts
- Try not to eat the same fruits and vegetables every day

Breads, other cereals and potatoes
What counts?
This food group, sometimes referred to as 'starchy carbohydrates', includes bread, potatoes (including low fat oven chips), yams, breakfast cereals,

pasta, rice, oats, noodles, maize, millet and cornmeal.

How much should you eat?
Most of us should eat more!

Base a third of your food intake on foods from this group, aiming to include at least one food from this group at each meal, e.g. potatoes with fish and vegetables, a chicken salad sandwich, stir-fried vegetables with rice, or porridge oats for breakfast.

Potatoes, yams, plantains and sweet potato fall into this group, rather than fruit and vegetables, because they contain starchy carbohydrates.

Why eat these foods?
These foods provide:
Carbohydrate: a source of energy
Fibre: keeps the gut healthy and helps prevent constipation
Some calcium: required for the development and maintenance of healthy bones
Some iron: needed for healthy red blood cells
B vitamins: e.g. thiamin and niacin – which help the body use energy
Folate:* needed for red blood cells

Healthy eating tips
- Base your meals around foods from this group
- Eat wholegrain or wholemeal breads, pastas and cereals as well as white choices
- Choose low fat oven chips rather than fried chips (oven chips fall into this food group but fried chips don't)
- Eating more foods from this group will help to reduce the proportion of fat and increase the amount of fibre in the diet
- Avoid frying or adding too much fat to these foods

Milk and dairy foods
What counts?
This food group includes milk, cheese, yogurt and fromage frais. Calcium fortified soya alternatives to milk can also be included. This group does not include butter, eggs and cream as these fall into other food groups.

How much should you eat?
Eat moderate amounts.

Try to eat 2-3 servings a day. A serving of milk is a 200ml glass, a

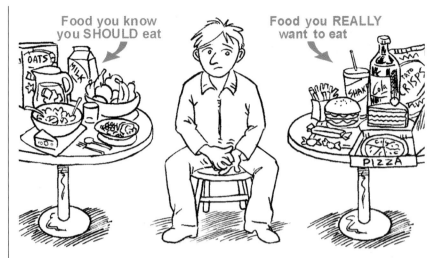

Food you know you SHOULD eat

Food you REALLY want to eat

serving of yogurt is a small pot (150g), a serving of cheese is 30g (matchbox size). Choose lower fat versions whenever you can, such as semi-skimmed milk, low fat yogurt and reduced fat cheese.

Healthy eating tips
- Choose low fat milk i.e. semi-skimmed or skimmed milk
- Choose low fat yogurts and reduced fat cheeses

Why eat these foods?
These foods provide:
Calcium: needed for development and maintenance of healthy bones
Zinc: required for tissue growth and repair
Protein: needed for growth and repair, and also a source of energy
Vitamin B12: required for blood cells and nerve function
Vitamin B2: needed for the release of energy from carbohydrates and protein
Vitamin A: (in whole milk products) for growth, development and eyesight

Meat, fish and alternatives
What counts?
This food group includes meat, poultry, fish, eggs and alternatives (see below). Meat products include bacon, salami, sausages, beefburgers and paté. Fish includes frozen and canned fish such as sardines and tuna, fish fingers and fish cakes.

How much should you eat?
Eat moderate amounts.

Choose lower fat versions whenever you can. Some meat products, e.g. beefburgers and

sausages, can be high in fat. Trim visible fat off meat where possible. The Government recommends that we eat two portions of fish each week, one of which should be an oily fish (e.g. salmon, mackerel, trout, sardines or fresh tuna).

Alternatives
These include nuts, tofu, myco-protein, textured vegetable protein (TVP), beans such as kidney beans and canned baked beans, and pulses such as lentils. These foods provide protein, fibre and iron but unlike those listed above are not a rich source of zinc and generally provide no vitamin B12 (unless fortified).

Why eat these foods?
These foods provide:
Protein: needed for growth and repair, also a source of energy
Iron: especially red meat, needed for healthy red blood cells
B Vitamins: especially vitamin B12
Vitamin D: in meat, required for healthy bones
Zinc: required for tissue growth and repair
Magnesium: helps the body use energy. Needed for healthy tissues and bones
Omega-3 fatty acids: in oily fish, may help protect against heart disease

Healthy eating tips
- Choose lower fat meat products
- Choose lean cuts of meat
- Cut visible fat including skin from meat and poultry and drain away fat after cooking
- Try to grill, roast or microwave meat and fish rather than frying
- Eat oily fish once a week

Foods containing fat and foods containing sugar

Foods containing fat: what counts?
Margarine, butter, other spreading fats and low fat spreads, cooking oils, oil-based salad dressings, mayonnaise, cream, fried foods including fried chips, chocolate, crisps, biscuits, pastries, cake, puddings, ice cream, rich sauces and gravies are all in this food group because they contain fat.

Foods containing sugar: what counts?
Soft drinks (not diet drinks), sweets, jam and sugar, as well as foods such as cakes, puddings, biscuits, pastries and ice cream.

How much should you eat?
Most people need to eat less!

It is essential to have a small amount of fat in the diet, but eat foods containing fat sparingly as they are high in energy. Look out for reduced fat or low fat alternatives (by law any food labelled as low fat must contain no more than 3g of fat per 100g). Fats can be divided into saturates, monounsaturates and polyunsaturates.

Limit consumption of saturates, associated with animal products, cakes, biscuits and pastries, to reduce risk of heart disease. To cut down on saturates, make use of the information on nutrition panels on food products, cut off visible fat from meat and poultry, choose lower fat meat and dairy products, and where fat is needed in cooking use it sparingly.

Choose fats and oils containing monounsaturates (e.g. olive and rapeseed oils) and polyunsaturates (e.g. sunflower, corn and rapeseed oils) instead of saturates. In moderation these are not associated with an increased risk of heart disease – but still use them sparingly. There are two types of essential fats, which must be supplied by the diet in small amounts: omega-3 fatty acids (e.g. found in oily fish, walnuts, omega-3 enriched eggs, and rapeseed and soya oil) and omega-6 fatty acids (e.g. found in vegetable oils such as sunflower, corn and soya oil and spreads made from these).

Sugar adds flavour and sweetness to foods, but frequent consumption of sugar-containing foods and drinks is associated with an increased tendency towards tooth decay.

Healthy eating tips
- Eat small quantities of these foods
- Choose low fat or reduced sugar foods where possible
- Use spreads and oils sparingly – opt for vegetable fats and oils
- Try to limit consumption of sugar-containing foods and drinks between meals
- Try not to add fat to foods when cooking

What about salt?
Salt is needed for the body to function properly. However, many of us consume much more than is needed. The Government recommends that the average intake of salt should be reduced by a third to 6g/day for adults; less for children. Choose foods that are low in salt, and try to avoid adding salt to foods during cooking and at the table. Sodium is often labelled on foods rather than salt – to roughly convert sodium to salt simply multiply the sodium figure by 2.5.

What about supplements?
For most healthy people, a varied and balanced diet will provide all the vitamins and minerals the body needs. There are certain times in our lives when we may benefit from taking supplements but remember supplements cannot replace a healthy diet. If you think that your diet is not meeting your nutrient requirements, a multivitamin and mineral supplement may be of benefit. Avoid supplements with high doses of single vitamins or minerals as these may well be unnecessary and should not be taken without seeking medical advice.

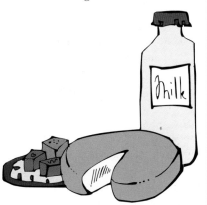

What about fluids?
The amount of fluid we need varies from person to person – age, climate, diet and physical activity all have an influence. Intakes of 1.5 to 2 litres of fluids a day are recommended in temperate climates and this includes water and other drinks like squash, fruit juices, tea and coffee. Some of our fluid requirement comes from the food we eat, rather than drinks – this counts too.

What about alcohol?
Drink sensibly! This means a maximum of 3-4 units per day for men and 2-3 units per day for women. A unit is 25ml of spirits (standard pub measure), 125ml (small glass) of wine or half a pint of standard strength lager, beer or cider. Drinking more than recommended can have adverse effects on your health. Avoid binge drinking in particular.

What about pregnancy?
Pregnant women should follow a healthy balanced diet at all times, however specific dietary advice exists with regards to a number of foods.

What about phytochemicals?
Phytochemicals, also known as bioactive substances, are compounds commonly found in plant foods that are not considered to be nutrients but may have beneficial effects on health, helping to protect against a number of diseases such as heart disease and cancer.

* Folic acid (400µg/day) supplements (a form of folate) are recommended for women of childbearing age, up until the 12th week of pregnancy. See www.nutrition.org.uk/healthyeating.htm for more information.

- This information is intended for all healthy individuals over the age of 5 years.

Further information on topics covered in this article is available from www.nutrition.org.uk/healthyeating.htm, or contact us at British Nutrition Foundation, High Holborn House, 52-54 High Holborn, London, WC1V 6RQ. www.nutrition.org.uk
© *British Nutrition Foundation, 2004*

A balanced diet

Healthy eating means getting a wide variety of the right foods into your diet. A balanced diet is not rigid or miserable, and has room in it for the occasional treat

What nutrients do you need?

To keep running smoothly, your body needs:

- Carbohydrates (sugars and starchy food), for energy
- Proteins, for building muscle etc.
- Fats, for energy and making cell walls, etc.
- Fibre, to keep the gut healthy
- Vitamins and minerals, for a wide range of functions
- Water, to flush out the waste products of your metabolism

Getting the balance right

- Eat regular meals based on carbohydrate in the form of unrefined starchy foods. This means potatoes in their skins, rice, bread and pasta. The wholemeal versions are the best as they are thought to contain more vitamins and release their energy more steadily, as well as containing fibre.
- Refined sugary food can cause tooth decay and cause fluctuations in blood glucose levels. Sugar is 'empty calories' and contains only energy without other nutrients (the same goes for alcohol).
- Protein is needed in moderate amounts. Go for lean meats,

TheSite.org

poultry, eggs, fish, beans, lower-fat cheeses, semi-skimmed milk, yogurts, or soya products.

- Fats are essential to health in small amounts. You need roughly equal amounts of saturates (e.g. butter), monounsaturates (e.g. olive oil) and polyunsaturates (e.g. sunflower oil). Try to avoid hardened vegetable oils as they usually contain trans fatty acids that are unhealthy forms of fat.
- Vitamins and minerals are best obtained from eating a wide variety of foods. The ones in the tablets (and added to fortified cereals etc.) are often not in the same natural forms that are found in food, and may not be absorbed as effectively. Try to eat at least five portions of different kinds of fruit or veg every day to stay in top condition.
- Eat breakfast and don't skip meals. You'll be more alert and your metabolism will be better. People who eat breakfast regularly are more likely to be slim than people who skip it.

- Combine a balanced diet with regular moderate exercise to feel and look your best.
- Make friends with food, it isn't the enemy. It's there to be enjoyed. If you eat something unhealthy, try not to feel guilty, just aim to eat more healthily the next day.

If you stick to these guidelines most of the time, it will be fine if you occasionally eat small amounts of sweet foods and fried foods.

Do you really need to lose weight?

You need to look up your body mass index (BMI), which is a formula that takes into account both your height and your weight. It will give you a healthy range of weights, there isn't a single correct weight to be for your height. Go to your doctor to be weighed and measured, and ask her or him for some medical advice about weight loss. The bathroom scales at home are not accurate enough to give you an exact reading of how much you weigh.

- The above information is taken from TheSite.org website. TheSite.org aims to offer the best guide to life for young adults, aged 16-25.

© TheSite.org

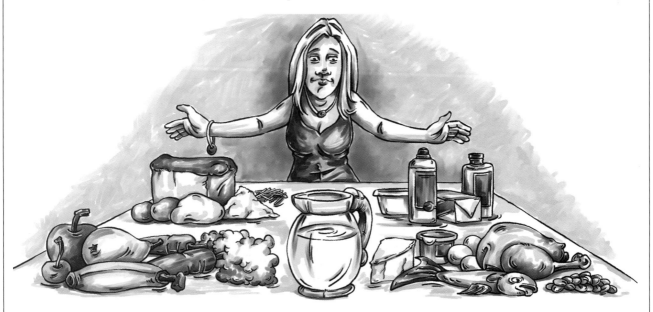

Junk food timebomb

The junk food timebomb that threatens a new generation. The Government's top food adviser has issued a shock warning that life expectancy could fall if Britain does not tackle the obesity problem. Jo Revill and Kamal Ahmed reveal the latest fears over our ever growing waistlines

Trailing down a Sainsbury superstore aisle, Debbie Oakley, 46-year-old mother of three, wore a glazed expression as she surveyed the range of cereals. Her six-year-old son, Matthew, began to clamour for two packets with free toys inside, and into the trolley they went. The sugary contents didn't seem to matter. It was Friday evening and she wanted to get home to cook dinner.

'If you've got young children and you work, you can't read the labelling because you haven't got time,' confessed Oakley, a secretary with a Bristol firm. 'If they package it clearly, then I don't mind, but if it has small print, then I don't have time to read the labels.'

She admits that her 16- and 18-year-old children still avoid the vegetables on their plate and fears that her youngest is heading the same way. 'Matthew picks things with lots of sugar and it's hard to get them to eat something without a sugar coating.'

So how much responsibility does Oakley bear for her children's health – and how much lies with the food giants who make billions pandering to the appetites of the young Matthews of this world for fatty, sugary, salty food? The battle over what we put in our trollies is rapidly becoming one of the most perplexing issues taxing the Government, which faces an unprecedented obesity epidemic. There has never been, in the space of a single generation, such a dramatic deterioration in public health caused by a single phenomenon. The twin evils of junk food and inactivity will inevitably leave thousands of Britons with disabilities, but diabetes and arthritis are the least of their problems. Fat people tend to die prematurely.

Obesity now affects 21 per cent of men and 23 per cent of women in the UK. A further 46 per cent of men and 33 per cent of women are overweight. At least two-thirds of our population needs to shed pounds – the exact opposite of a century ago when the same proportion of Britons were underweight through lack of nutrition. As for children, one in 25 is now classified as obese.

Nor is this an issue for the Western world alone. China now has 20 million diabetics, many of whom have sunk into chronic ill health and the prospect of an early grave as a result of abandoning their traditional diet of rice, fish and green vegetables. The Greeks, who pride themselves on their olive oil and fresh salads, nevertheless have high rates of obesity in children, who opt instead for hamburgers. The World Health Organisation has identified being overweight as a global problem, pointing out that more than 300 million people are obese. It is astonishing that in the space of a single generation non-communicable diseases, such as heart problems, diabetes, cancer and respiratory illness, now account for more deaths each year around the globe than infections such as HIV and malaria. We are eating ourselves to death.

Obesity now affects 21 per cent of men and 23 per cent of women in the UK. A further 46 per cent of men and 33 per cent of women are overweight

---

With obesity come metabolic changes which human physiology was never designed to withstand. Blood pressure rises, as do cholesterol levels and insulin resistance. The joints, particularly knee joints, have extra strain placed on them. Women become less fertile and men find it harder to sleep because breathing is more laboured.

The likelihood of developing Type 2 diabetes rises as the pounds go on. Around 85 per cent of the world's diabetics are Type 2, and 90 per cent of them are overweight. America and Britain have high rates but will be overtaken, if trends continue, by India and the Middle East within two decades.

Britain should be well placed to counteract this international medical phenomenon, with its national health service and strong tradition of public health measures aimed at helping the poorest. But how far can the Government go in regulating the food industry and coercing parents into giving children proper meals and lots of exercise? The man who must confront this problem is Sir John Krebs, chairman of the Food Standards Agency. Krebs has to tell Britain how it should tackle its 'ticking timebomb', as he describes it.

This weekend he has outlined a number of options in the agency's first report. Should advertising directed at children for sweets and high-fat foods be controlled? Should schools ban vending machines dispensing sugary drinks, salty snacks and sweets? Should companies be stopped from setting up promotions with schools to encourage children to buy more sweets (Cadbury's) or crisps (Walker's) in return for new sports equipment or books?

'If nothing is done to stop the trend, for the first time in 100 years life expectancy will actually go down,' Krebs warned. 'We increasingly rely on food prepared by others – that's just a fact of life nowadays when a lot of families are two working parents in a hurry.'

Krebs worries about how you enable people like Oakley to make the choices she needs to make. 'Our research shows that people would like some simple signposts. At the moment it might say on a chocolate bar that it contains so many kilo-joules. What the hell do you and I know about kilojoules? If it said this is high or medium or low [in fat or sugar] that might be more helpful.'

But already the Food and Drink Federation, representing the industry, is going on the defensive. It issued a vehement press release: 'Parents will take a dim view of any "Nanny State" type approaches to matters of personal choice. With an average UK supermarket offering some 30,000 products, the terms "healthier foods" and "less healthy foods" are meaningless in the context of a healthy balanced diet.'

Yet the public is clearly growing more distrustful of the way food is produced and the marketing devices used, such as the 'super-sizing' of chocolate bars, to sell more and more products.

This weekend Sainsbury's will announce a drive to cut salt in its products. Salt matters as much as sugar and fat because excessive amounts cause thousands of heart attacks and strokes each year. Sainsbury's three-year drive will see levels reduced in pizzas, soups and sandwiches, but not by nearly enough to satisfy the physicians.

Professor Graham MacGregor, head of cardiovascular medicine of St George's Hospital Medical School, said an immediate cut of 10 per cent in salt in the average diet would save 5,800 lives over the next year and is unhappy that this is not being forced upon manufacturers. 'The industry tells us that they can't cut salt levels immediately because the customers won't like the taste, but lots of studies show that such a reduction wouldn't be detectable. I find it astonishing that a train operator can be held accountable if he causes deaths in a rail crash but we don't hold the manufacturers responsible for these many thousands of preventable deaths because so much salt is hidden in processed food.'

At a meeting public health Minister Melanie Johnson will push for further cuts in salt levels, yet her position typifies the Government's strange relationship with the industry. She will call on them to do more, warning that they have until February to show progress. Yet the Government is reluctant to impose regulations on an industry which is so powerful. All the talk is of voluntary codes, not compulsory rules.

Meanwhile the Health Select Committee, an influential group of MPs, is holding its own inquiry into obesity. In two weeks' time it will summon the heads of the major food corporations. Julian Hilton-Johnson, vice-president of McDonald's, Martin Glenn, president of PepsiCo UK, and Andrew Cosslett, managing director of Cadbury Schweppes, will sit in a row in front of the committee to explain why they are not responsible for the surge in obesity.

One of the MPs questioning them will be Paul Burstow, Lib Dem spokesman on health. Last month he flew with the rest of the committee to Coca-Cola's headquarters in Atlanta, Georgia. 'They had gone to the trouble of bringing in a dietitian from California, who gave us a mantra about how exercise was the problem. My jaw dropped as I listened to her. The idea that you can burn off all the calories from a high-fat diet just through exercise is potty. I hope in our next meeting that the companies will put forward some solutions.'

Many people think of obesity as akin to smoking, both being major causes of chronic illness, disability and early death, and both seen as the creation of marketing men who have learnt to indulge our cravings. But whereas even one cigarette is harmful to the body, the same cannot be said for a chocolate bar or burger. Obesity expert Dr Susan Jebb points out: 'No one food, in itself, is dangerous – it is a prolonged excessive amount of high-fat, high-sugar food which creates the problems.'

We live in what nutritionists call an obesifying environment. Some people are genetically more predisposed to weight gain than others, but the food has to be available in the first place. As one

Food and drinks consumed

Proportion of all children, aged 4 to 18, consuming foods and drinks over 7-day period by sex

Food group	Food	Boys	Girls
Fruit and vegetables	Baked beans	62	57
	Leafy green vegetables	39	44
	Raw and salad vegetables	47	59
	Citrus fruits	24	28
	Bananas	38	38
Bread, other cereals and potatoes	Pasta	60	64
	Rice	42	40
	White bread	95	96
	Wholemeal bread	22	26
	Chips	89	88
Meat, fish and alternatives	Bacon and ham	61	57
	Burgers and kebabs	41	35
	Sausages	64	55
	Meat pies and pastries	46	43
	Chicken and turkey dishes	75	73
	Coated and fried white fish	49	44
	Eggs	45	44
Milk and dairy foods	Whole milk	54	51
	Semi-skimmed milk	59	57
	Cheese (excl. cottage cheese)	65	69
	Yogurt	40	44
Fats and sugars	Biscuits	84	84
	Buns, cakes and pastries	76	75
	Ice cream	51	50
	Chocolate confectionery	84	80
Drinks	Fruit juice	46	51
	Carbonated soft drinks not low calorie	78	75
	Concentrated soft drinks not low calorie	52	51

Source: National Diet and Nutrition Survey: young people aged 4 to 18 years. Office for National Statistics, March 2004

expert put it: 'If your genes load the gun, then it's your environment that's pulling the trigger.' And in a world where food is cheaper and more accessible than ever, a moderate consumption becomes increasingly hard to achieve.

The issue plagues all Ministers, especially Culture Secretary Tessa Jowell, who now has to decide whether to do more to ban food adverts targeted at children. 'All the efforts have to be driven by a profound cultural change,' she said. 'We all cut corners, we all buy processed food. Now we have to identify the areas that are the role of government and those that are for industry and those to do with parental behaviour.'

A major aim is to raise levels of physical activity, and Jowell has seen many schools where they are trying to do this: 'I have seen the impact in areas where they have brought in partnerships,' she said. *The Observer*, as part of its Fit for the Future campaign, has argued that all children need two hours of sport in school each week, but many schools are unable to offer even that. Jowell said parents can help: 'You have to persuade them of the value of taking children to sport on a Saturday morning. If they won't do that, you have to look at offering sport before school or more sport after school. But there's a lot of pressure on teachers, so we want to get more coaches to come in and help.'

And as if anyone needed reminding, she said: 'It takes a long time to secure change. It's not going to happen overnight.'

The facts about flab

- One in 40 women in the UK is now morbidly obese, meaning that their health is at very serious risk from their weight.
- In Thailand, 15 per cent of children are obese, up from 12 per cent just two years ago.

- In Chinese cities, one in five adults is now obese.
- It takes one-and-a-half hours of running to burn off the calories contained in a supersized Mars bar.
- A boy aged eight is the ideal customer for soft drinks companies, according to an industry journal, as he has 65 years of consumption ahead of him.
- Coca-Cola increased its sales by 7 per cent in 2001 when it teamed up with Warner to promote the film *Harry Potter and the Philosopher's Stone*.
- Almost £452m was spent on food advertising in the UK last year. McDonald's spent £42m of it.
- More than half the world's population fails to do 30 minutes of moderate activity a day.

- This article first appeared in *The Observer*, 9 November 2003.

© *The Observer*

New food bill to combat child obesity

A fresh attempt to help tackle childhood obesity through legislation is being launched. Debra Shipley MP is due to present a Private Member's Bill in the House of Commons aimed at improving children's diets.

The Bill would require the Food Standards Agency to specify criteria for healthy and unhealthy foods, taking into account nutritional content and use of additives.

The criteria would then be used for a ban on marketing unhealthy foods at children.

The Children's Food Bill also requires new regulations to improve school meals, demands practical food skills be included in the National Curriculum, and seeks a ban on the sale of unhealthy foods in school vending machines.

Advertising ban

Ms Shipley, Labour MP for Stourbridge, introduced a Bill last year calling for a ban on advertising of food and drink high in fat, salt or sugar during children's television. It failed after running out of parliamentary time.

'Obesity has doubled in six-year-olds and trebled among 15-year-olds over a 10-year period,' Ms Shipley said.

'As a consequence, adult-onset diabetes is now being seen in schoolchildren.

'It is not surprising that the Chief Medical Officer has described the problem as a "public health time bomb" that needs to be defused.

'It is no longer good enough to hold consultations, produce reviews and call on the industry to mend its ways. Action is urgently needed.

'This Bill will bring forward a wide range of measures to tackle the childhood obesity epidemic and improve children's diet-related health.'

Children's Food Bill

The Children's Food Bill has been developed by Sustain, the food and farming alliance, with support from 114 national organisations including the British Heart Foundation, Cancer Research UK, Friends of the Earth, Royal College of General Practitioners and the National Union of Teachers.

Charlie Powell, project officer at Sustain, said: 'As huge profits are at stake, calls for the junk food industry to act voluntarily are simply naive.

'Our coalition of 114 national organisations recognises that statutory measures to improve children's diets are urgently needed.'

- This article first appeared in the *Daily Mail*, 18 May 2004.

© *2004 Associated Newspapers Ltd*

How to be a healthy weight

Information from the Food Standards Agency

If you have any concerns about your weight, contact your GP or a dietitian. If you think you just need to lose a little weight, here are some practical tips. You might want to look at ways of:

- only eating as much food as you need
- improving the balance of your diet
- getting more active

Whenever we eat more than our body needs, we put on weight. This is because our body stores the energy we don't use up, usually as fat. Even small amounts of surplus energy each day can lead to weight gain.

Getting the balance right

It's not a good idea to go on a crash diet and it's important to make sure you continue to eat a balanced diet. Otherwise you might not be getting all the nutrients you need to keep your body healthy.

When you're trying to make a healthy choice, for most people, the aim should be to:

- cut down on fat – especially saturates
- eat more fruit and vegetables
- eat more starchy foods such as bread, pasta and rice
- cut down on salt and sugar

Fruit and veg should make up a third of the food you eat. Aim to eat at least five portions every day, and these can be fresh, frozen, tinned, dried or cooked, and a glass of fruit juice can also make up one of your portions each day. As a guide, a portion means:

- one apple or banana
- two smaller fruit such as plums
- two to three tablespoonfuls of vegetables

It's best to vary the types of fruit and veg you eat so that you increase the range and proportion of the different nutrients in your diet.

Starchy foods should also make up about a third of your diet. These include:

- bread
- breakfast cereals
- pasta
- rice
- potatoes
- beans and lentils

Try to eat a variety of these foods and choose wholegrain, wholemeal or 'high fibre' varieties whenever possible.

Whenever we eat more than our body needs, we put on weight. This is because our body stores the energy we don't use up, usually as fat

---

You might think that starchy foods are particularly fattening. But this isn't true, although they can become fattening if they're cooked or served with added fat. It's the margarine or butter we spread on bread, the cream or cheese sauce we add to pasta, or the oil we use for frying, that makes them fattening.

A healthy diet means eating and drinking less fat and sugar.

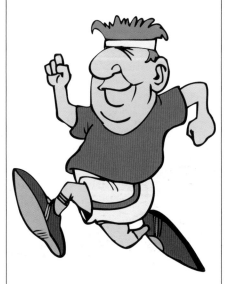

You'll probably eat some foods containing fat every day, such as margarine or butter, cooking oils, oil-based salad dressings and mayonnaise, but keep these to small amounts and choose low fat varieties where possible.

And there's no escaping the fact that you should keep cakes, biscuits, crisps, pastries and ice cream to a minimum. And remember to choose low-fat alternatives when you can.

If you make changes to the types of foods you eat and the way you cook them, this might help you to adopt long-term healthy eating patterns for the future. For example, you could try to:

- fill up on bread, cereals, potatoes and fruit and veg
- choose lean cuts of meat and always trim off any fat
- choose lower-fat varieties of dairy foods such as semi-skimmed or skimmed milk, reduced-fat cheese, lower-fat yogurts
- boil, steam, grill, poach or microwave food rather than frying or roasting

Getting physical

Physical activity is a good way of using up extra calories, and helps us to maintain our body weight. It's a good idea to get active each day, but you don't need to join a gym if you don't want to. Here are some suggestions of activities that will help you to burn off excess energy. You could:

- go for a walk after lunch
- choose the stairs instead of taking the lift
- walk (or even jog) some of your shorter journeys
- get off the bus one or two stops earlier

- The above information is from the Government's Food Standards Agency's website which can be found at www.foodstandards.gov.uk

Food quality and your health

Information from the Soil Association

Is organic food more nutritious?

More nutrients and less water
Artificial fertilisers increase the water content of fruit and vegetables. Although this method may produce bigger yields, it dilutes the nutrient content of fruit and vegetables.

More minerals and more vitamin C
Research comparing the nutrient contents of organic and non-organic fruit and vegetables reveals a strong trend toward higher levels in organic produce. Of 27 valid comparisons of the mineral and vitamin C contents of organic and non-organic crops, 14 showed significantly higher levels in organic produce while just one favoured non-organic.

More protective antioxidants in organic produce
Plants contain some 5,000–10,000 naturally occurring compounds (known as phytonutrients) that are often involved in protecting the plant from pests and diseases. Because organic crops are not artificially protected with pesticides they tend to produce more naturally occurring phytonutrients, many of which are now known to have protective

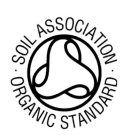

(antioxidant) properties. Some are proving useful in the prevention and treatment of cancer.

Is organic food better for you?

The Soil Association has always maintained that health cannot be defined as simply the absence of disease but rather a profound state of well-being and vitality. While considerable improvements have occurred in disease treatment, serious concerns about our overall health persist due to increases in allergies, infertility, and many diseases including cancer.

So can organic food, with fewer toxins and more nutrients, make a difference to our health?
Clinical and observational evidence in humans suggests that it can, although it's difficult to do controlled studies with people because of

complicating factors like genes and lifestyle. In controlled animal feeding trials, however, the evidence is clear – animals fed organically produced feed are healthier in terms of growth, reproductive health and recovery from illness than those fed on non-organic feed, even over successive generations.

Is organic food safer?

Organic food contains fewer pesticide residues
Pesticide residues are rarely found on organic food. In contrast, pesticides are found on one in three non-organic foods tested each year, and multiple residues of up to seven different compounds are not uncommon. Pesticide safety is tested for individual compounds, but we know very little about the 'cocktail effect' of multiple residues. Some research suggests that they may be hundreds of times more toxic than the same compounds individually.

Organic food contains fewer food additives
While food manufacturers can use more than 500 additives, organic food processors are prohibited from using a host of ingredients that researchers say may be harmful to our health

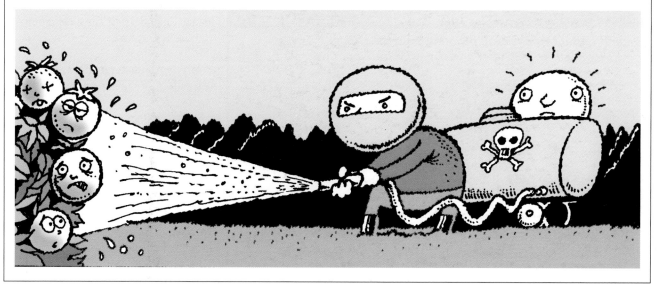

such as aspartame, hydrogenated fat, phosphoric acid, sulphur dioxide, monosodium glutamate, or artificial flavourings and colourings.

Organically born and reared cattle are BSE-free

Applying common sense and the precautionary principle, organic farming banned the feeding of animal protein to farm animals well before the BSE crisis hit UK agriculture. The Soil Association has found no recorded cases of BSE in any animal born and reared organically.

Organic farming bans GMOs

There is insufficient evidence to prove that genetically modified organisms (GMOs) are safe, and some animal feeding trials have revealed unexpected toxicities.

Organic farming cuts antibiotic use

Antibiotics are used extensively in non-organic farming to promote growth and to prevent disease in intensively reared, overcrowded farm animals. High standards of animal welfare in organic farming minimise the need for antibiotics and other veterinary drugs which are used only when strictly necessary.

Organic standards minimise food poisoning risks

A recent government survey gave organic food a clean bill of health and confirmed expectations that organic methods, such as the careful composting of manure, minimise pathogenic risks such as E.coli o157.

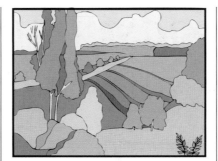

'There is a continuing threat to human health from imprudent use of antibiotics in animals'

House of Lords select committee

How does organic farming produce healthier food?

Healthy plants, animals and people depend on healthy soil.

Organic farming nurtures soil life

A gram of soil contains millions of micro-organisms too small to see, and some of them are now known to work with plants to help provide more nutrients. Research has shown that organically managed soil receiving compost and manure can have up to 85% more healthy soil life than that bombarded with chemical fertilisers and pesticides.

Organic farming returns nutrients to the soil

Plants remove up to 60 minerals from the soil but non-organic farmers usually replace only those necessary for plant growth – nitrogen, phosphorus and potassium (NPK). Over time this can lead to depletion of all the other minerals. Organic farmers use manures and composts containing a wide variety of minerals and not just NPK, so deficiencies are less likely to develop.

Organic farming rotates crops

Growing the same crops each year in the same soil can lead to depletion of the nutrients used by that crop, so organic farmers rotate their crops and include 'green manures' in the rotation – crops that fix nitrogen from the air into the soil, allow the soil to rest, and at the end of the season are ploughed back in. All this helps prevent the soil from becoming minerally depleted, so it can go on producing healthy crops.

Action!

Vote with your fork

Buy organically produced food wherever possible. This sends a clear message to retailers and the government about your preference for organic food.

Write to your MP

Ask her or him to write to the Minister for Public Health at the Department of Health, Richmond House, 79 Whitehall, London SW1A 2NL.

Ask your MP to represent your view that the Food Standards Agency should commission adequate research to investigate comparative differences between non-organic and organic food. Please send us copies of your letters and any replies.

Read the evidence for yourself

Previous reviews of this type have failed to screen out the many studies of poor quality that did not properly represent organic food or farming. Buy the Soil Association's latest and most thorough report – *Organic Farming, Food Quality and Human Health* – by nutritionist Shane Heaton, and assess the evidence for yourself.

'Any conclusion upon the safety of introducing genetically modified materials into the UK is premature as there is insufficient evidence to inform the decision-making process at the moment.'

British Medical Association

■ The above information is from the Soil Association. For further information visit their website: www.soilassociation.org

© Soil Association 2000-2004

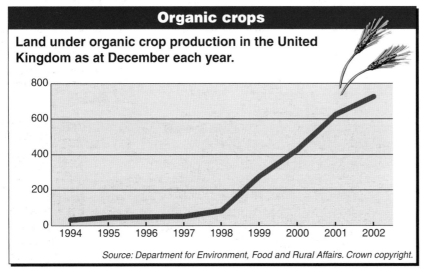

Organic crops

Land under organic crop production in the United Kingdom as at December each year.

Source: Department for Environment, Food and Rural Affairs. Crown copyright.

Is breakfast important?

Information from the British Nutrition Foundation

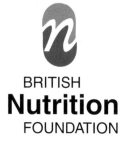

BRITISH Nutrition FOUNDATION

Yes! Breakfast is important for a number of reasons:

- Overnight our bodies need energy, even while we are asleep. In particular, the brain needs glucose (a form of carbohydrate). Carbohydrate is supplied from the day's meals and snacks and is stored as glycogen in our muscles and liver. So overnight some of our glycogen is broken down into glucose and used by the body as energy. We need to eat breakfast to replace some of the glycogen stores and to provide energy for the morning's activities.

- Another reason for having a breakfast is the so-called kick-start it gives to our metabolic rate. After every meal there is a surge in oxygen uptake as food is digested and absorbed. This is associated with an increase in heat production and so is more commonly known as the thermic effect of feeding. Overnight while you have been asleep, your metabolism slows down, so eating soon after you wake up helps boost your metabolism and gets the body going again.

- That's not all, research has shown that skipping the first meal of the day may lead to an unhealthy pattern of snacking on high-fat foods throughout the morning. This is particularly true for children who leave the house on an empty stomach and stop to buy sweets and crisps on the way to school.

Breakfast is a great way to get plenty of the essential nutrients that the body needs each day. There is even research to show that people who eat breakfast are more likely to have more nutritionally balanced diets, that are lower in fat and higher in carbohydrate compared to those who miss breakfast. Eating cereal for breakfast, which is low in fat and high in carbohydrate, promotes the feeling of being full for longer so reducing mid-morning cravings for fatty snacks. Fortified breakfast cereals also provide important vitamins such as the B vitamins (necessary for energy production) and minerals such as iron (necessary for healthy blood). Milk is an important source of protein, B vitamins such as riboflavin and B12, and minerals such as zinc, magnesium and particularly calcium (necessary for healthy bones and teeth).

There is a small amount of evidence to show that academic performance can be boosted by a high-energy breakfast. Overnight blood sugar levels drop and can be low on waking. Studies have linked low blood sugar levels to poor memory, concentration and learning. Eating breakfast raises blood sugar levels and helps us to function more effectively.

Research has also been conducted to see if there is a link between iron in the diet and IQ. Some of these studies have demonstrated a possible positive association between IQ scores and iron intake. Iron intake is important, particularly in young women, and breakfast foods provide a good opportunity to provide iron-containing foods such as wholegrain cereals and breads and yeast extract spread. A glass of orange juice will provide vitamin C, which is necessary for the absorption of iron from non-meat sources.

The consumption of wholegrain foods also offers other advantages to general health and well-being. Research has shown that people with a lower risk of diseases such as heart disease and some cancers tend to eat more wholegrain foods as part of a healthy lifestyle. A diet high in fibre is recommended to promote good bowel health.

Breakfast is one of the easiest meals in which to get calcium into the diet through the consumption of milk and dairy products such as yogurt. A serving of milk on cereal can provide up to half our daily calcium requirement.

- The above information is from the British Nutrition Foundation's website which can be found at www.nutrition.org.uk

© British Nutrition Foundation 2004

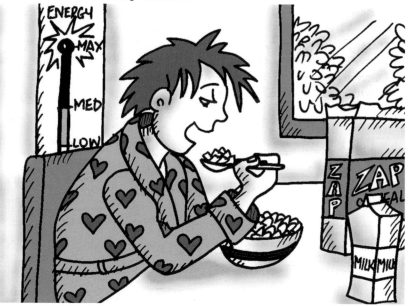

Salt and health

Information from the the British Dietetic Association. By Luci Daniels RD

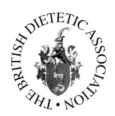

The problem

Eating too much salt can increase your risk of developing high blood pressure. High blood pressure is linked to heart disease and strokes. By reducing your salt intake it is possible to reduce your blood pressure and your risk of developing heart problems, so it's well worth doing.

A lot of foods are not obviously salty, but do contain high amounts of 'hidden salt'. It's easier to make healthier food choices if you are able to quickly check the salt content on food labels.

How much?

The average salt intake is currently 9.5g a day (about 2 teaspoons), we should be having much less than this – the recommended intake is just 6g a day.

Salt in our diet comes from salt used in cooking, salt added at the table and salt added to processed foods. Surprisingly, about 75% of the salt we eat is already added to the food we buy.

Reducing your intake of salty processed foods is an important part of a healthy diet.

Salt sums

Salt is sodium chloride, and as food labels often list both salt and sodium content – it can be confusing.

To convert salt to sodium – divide by 2.5

To convert sodium to salt – multiply by 2.5

For example:
1g salt = 0.4g sodium
0.8g sodium = 2g salt

So what can you eat?

Fresh meat, fish, eggs, beans and lentils

Fruit and vegetables – including fresh, frozen, tinned without salt and juices

Cereals including rice, pasta, potatoes, bread, breakfast cereals and unsalted crackers

Milk, yogurt, soft white cheese [and small amounts of 'hard' cheese]

Fresh herbs, spices, pepper, vinegar, mustard, tomato purée

Let's be practical

Being realistic we all eat some processed or convenience foods most days. Choose lower salt options using the following guidelines:

For ready meals and sandwiches – choose meals with under 0.5g sodium per meal, that's 1.25g salt

For individual foods – soups, sauces, vegetables – choose foods with under 0.3g sodium per serving, that's 0.75g salt.

The main salty processed foods are:
- Salty meats such as ham, bacon, sausages, pâté
- Tinned, packet and instant soups
- Soy sauce, stock cubes, gravy powder and salted flavourings
- Any tinned food containing salt
- Smoked meat and fish
- Meat and yeast extracts

- Hard cheese [allowed 100g/4oz per week]
- Salted snacks like crisps, salted biscuits, popcorn
- High salt ready meals, sauces and take-away meals

Try to limit your intake of these salty foods to 1 serving a day.

Be salt aware

- Use a little salt in cooking.
- Try not to add extra salt at table.
- Cut right down on salty processed foods and ready meals.
- Check out food labels for salt and go for lower salt choices.

[If you have high blood pressure, being active, keeping a healthy weight, not drinking too much alcohol and regular check-ups are also important.]

- This Food Fact information is a public service of the British Dietetic Association intended for information only. It is not a substitute for proper medical diagnosis or dietary advice given by a Registered Dietitian (RD). To check that your dietitian is Registered check www.hpc-uk.org Other Food Fact sheets are available from www.bda.uk.com

© The British Dietetic Association
December 2003

Salt use

Use of salt in cooking and at the table by sex of respondent*

Use of salt in cooking and at the table**	Men	Women	All
Salt added to cooking			
usually added	71%	68%	68%
uses salt alternative	4%	6%	5%
not usually added	26%	27%	27%
Salt added at table			
usually	37%	28%	33%
occasionally	24%	23%	23%
rarely	15%	19%	17%
never	24%	30%	27%

* As reported in the dietary interview.
** Includes cases where salt alternative used.

Source: The National Diet & Nutrition Survey: adults aged 19 to 64 years. Crown copyright.

What is so good about fruit and vegetables?

Information from Sustain

Fruit and vegetables are excellent sources of vitamins, minerals and dietary fibre. In addition they provide other compounds with powerful disease reduction potential. There are over 100 of these substances and different types of fruit and vegetables are rich in different combinations. So our diets should include a wide variety of fruit and vegetables, particularly of different colours. There is also a displacement effect – that is, by eating more fruit and vegetables we tend to eat less of the fatty and sugary foods that are linked to obesity, heart disease, diabetes and tooth decay. Indeed, the evaluation of the Grab 5! pilot project showed that the increase in fruit and vegetable consumption was accompanied by a reduction in consumption of high fat snacks in some schools.

There is overwhelming evidence of the health benefits of eating fruit and vegetables, particularly in reducing the risks of heart disease, and some cancers. The World Cancer Research Fund estimates that diet and exercise could reduce cancer incidence by up to 40% and recent research has shown that children who eat the most fruit are 38% less likely to develop cancer in adulthood than those with the lowest intake.

The World Health Organisation recommends that we eat at least five portions a day. In the UK, on average people eat 2 or 3 portions, and children eat less than adults do. People on low incomes eat less fruit and vegetables than more affluent people, and are more likely to suffer from diet-related diseases.

Just about everyone in the UK should eat more fruit and vegetables. Schools can play a key role in encouraging children to eat more.

What is a portion?

An adult portion is 80g or 3 ounces or . . .

- one whole apple or orange
- a couple of kiwi fruits
- a helping of large fruit – melon, grapefruit, pineapple
- a handful of grapes or cherries
- a tablespoonful of raisins
- a bowl of salad
- two tablespoonsful of peas
- one corn on the cob
- a glass of fruit juice

Children's portions will be proportionately smaller. A good 'rule of thumb' is to think of a handful. The smaller (or bigger) the person's hand, the smaller (or bigger) the portion should be (a toddler's hand, a child's hand, a rugby player's hand etc.).

Fresh, frozen, dried and canned fruit and vegetables all count.

Juice and smoothies also count but only as one portion even if you drink more than one glass in a day.

Baked beans count as a portion but can only be counted once per day as can other pulses.

Potatoes do not count as a portion. They are included in the 'starchy staples' food group along with bread, rice and pasta.

Note that oral health advice is to limit consumption of dried fruits, juices and smoothies to meal times only to reduce the risks of tooth decay.

In 2002 the Department of Health launched a five a day campaign in England to encourage people to eat more fruit and vegetables.

Note that while take-aways, ready meals and several other food products may be marketed as contributing towards your 'five-a-day' because they contain some fruit or vegetables, they may also contain high amounts of sugar, fat and salt. Any health benefit from eating the fruit and vegetables is likely to be counterbalanced by the unhealthy levels of sugar, fat and/or salt also consumed. Always check the labels for the details.

- The above information is from Sustain's website which can be found at www.sustainweb.org

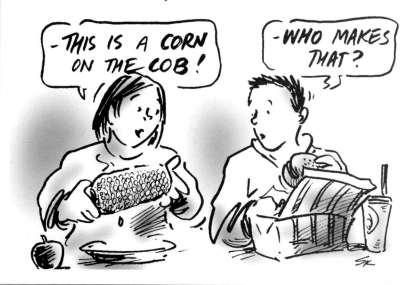

Four nutrition myths

Information from EUFIC

EUFIC

The Myth: Organic food is more nutritious

The Fact: Organic food is derived from crops or animals produced in a farming system that avoids the use of man-made fertilisers, pesticides, growth regulators and feed additives. Consumer attitude studies show that organic food consumption in Europe is part of a lifestyle, which results from an ideology, connected to a particular value system[1]. The view that organic foods are 'healthier' than conventionally produced foods appears to be based on the belief that organic foods have superior sensory attributes, contain lower levels of pesticides and synthetic fertilisers, and have higher levels of nutrients and protective phytochemicals. However, current evidence neither supports nor refutes the higher nutritional qualities attributed to organic food over conventionally produced food;[2] because nutritional quality and taste depend greatly on the variety and on growth conditions (e.g. soil, weather, etc.).

The Myth: Vegetarian diets are healthier than meat-based diets

The Fact: Vegetarian diets vary greatly and can range from avoiding meat through to a strict vegan diet, where all foods of animal origin are excluded. Some studies show that vegetarians suffer less from heart disease, some cancers, high blood pressure and type 2 diabetes, and that they live longer than meat-eaters. However, any beneficial effect is also likely to be due, in part, to a generally healthier lifestyle adopted by vegetarians including not smoking and taking more exercise.[3] It is not simply a case of omitting meat from the diet. Thus, a vegetarian diet is not automatically healthier than an omnivorous diet and non-vegetarians who are health conscious can live just as long as vegetarians. Vegetarian diets can even be unhealthy if meat and animal products, rich in essential vitamins (e.g. vit B12) and minerals (e.g. iron, zinc), are not substituted by nutritionally appropriate foods or compensated by adequate food supplements.

The Myth: Exercise is futile for weight control

The Fact: Despite the common view that an exercise-induced energy deficit will drive up hunger and energy intake, evidence shows this not to be the case, and that there is a role for exercise in weight loss and weight control.[4] So, why does physical activity often produce disappointing effects? Probably because of inappropriate food choices, a desire for self-reward after exercise, and a poor understanding of the relative rates at which energy can be expended by exercise, or taken in by eating. Therefore, diet and exercise (active lifestyle) should be considered jointly when managing your weight.

Exercise can also improve mood independent of age, gender and mode of exercise. It is now thought that psychological factors, such as perceived fitness, have a strong influence on exercise-induced mood changes. Thus, exercise is a behaviour that should be used to control body weight and improve mood.

The Myth: Food cravings indicate a nutrient deficiency

The Fact: A food craving is the desire to eat a specific food or type of food. Craving is experienced when attempts to restrict intake of certain foods cause the desire for that food to become more salient.[5] Women more commonly report food cravings than men do and in particular during the premenstrual phase, e.g. for choc-

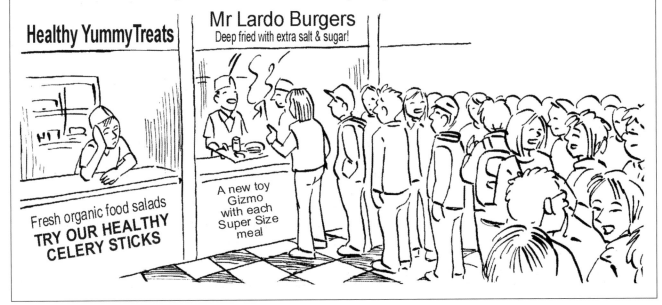

olate. Chocolate contains numerous pharmacological substances (e.g. caffeine, theobromine, phenylethylamine and anandamides) and minerals such as magnesium, which may contribute to improve premenstrual symptoms. However, the amounts present cannot explain the beneficial effects reported after consumption of chocolate. Therefore, attempts to self-regulate, for example, magnesium levels via chocolate consumption are not justified! A bar of chocolate contains only 50mg of magnesium whereas magnesium supplementation studies suggest over 1000mg are required to improve premenstrual symptoms. Thus, psychological factors (e.g. depressed mood, dissatisfaction with body image) are strong determinants of foods craved that tend to be high in fat and sweet-tasting, as these sensory attributes are perceived as providing emotional satisfaction.

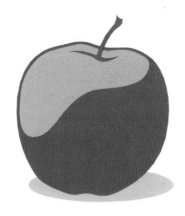

References

1. Risvik E, Issanchou S, Shepherd R & Tuorila H (2001) Measure-ments of consumer attitudes and their influence on food choice and acceptability (AIR-CAT). *Nutrition Metabolism and Cardio-vascular Disease* 11(4): 24-31. Summerbell C, Kelly, S & Campbell K. The prevention and treatment of childhood obesity. *Effective Health Care* Volume 7: Number 6, 2002.

2. Williams CM (2002) Nutritional quality of organic food: shades or grey or shades of green? *Proceedings of the Nutrition Society* 61: 19-24.
3. Dwyer J (1994) Vegetarian eating patterns: science, values, and food choices – where do we go from here? *American Journal of Clinical Nutrition* 59: S1255-S1262.
4. Blundell JE, King NA (1999) Physical activity and regulation of food intake: current evidence. *Med Sci Sports Exerc.* 31 (11 Suppl):S573-83.
5. Rogers PJ, Smit HJ (2000) Food craving and food 'addiction': a critical review of the evidence from a biopsychosocial per-spective. *Pharmacol Biochem Behav* 66(1):3-14.

■ The above information is from EUFIC's website which can be found at www.eufic.org

Food promotion to children

Agency agrees plan for an overhaul of the way food is promoted to children

The Board of the Food Standards Agency today (11 March 2004) agreed a series of far-reaching proposals to redress the imbalance of children's diets.

Sir John Krebs, Chair of the Food Standards Agency, said today: 'Children are bombarded with messages that promote food high in fat, salt and sugar. The evidence shows that these messages do influence children. Eating too much of these foods is storing up health problems for their future. The Food Standards Agency wants healthier choices to be promoted to children.

'Everyone has a responsibility to act and our action plan is a challenge to all with a part to play: not just parents and children, but Government, schools, the food and advertising industries and the celebrities and sporting heroes children look up to. Just because this is a complex issue doesn't mean we can't do anything about it.

'All parents are concerned about the health of their children; doing nothing to help them is not an option.'

The Action Plan commits the Agency to a range of initiatives, including:
■ developing advice and guidelines for the food industry on reducing amounts of fat, salt and sugar in products specifically aimed at children, and agreeing guidelines on the labelling of these products to enable consumers to identify more easily and accurately what are healthier options
■ monitoring food industry uptake of the Agency's advice and guidelines, and publishing the results for consumers to see what progress is being made
■ working with schools to push healthier foods higher up the menu. Targeting vending machines in schools to increase the range of healthier options
■ calling on celebrities to help redress the imbalance by promoting healthier food choices. This includes sports stars and sponsored events
■ working with broadcasters to encourage them to follow BBC Worldwide's initiative to increase the association between high profile characters and cartoons on TV and healthier foods
■ advising the broadcast regulator Ofcom, and the advertising industry, that action to address the imbalance in TV advertising of food to children is justified

■ The above information is from the Food Standards Agency's website which can be found at www.foodstandards.gov.uk

Parent power works!

BBC publishes nutrition policy… and Bob the Builder is shamed into action

BBC Worldwide, the commercial arm of the BBC, has published its long-awaited food and nutrition policy. This commits the BBC to use nutritional guidelines for the sorts of foods that can be promoted to children by means of its licensed pre-school characters such as the Teletubbies, Tweenies, Fimbles and Bill & Ben.

This development is a great victory for the Food Commission's Parents Jury. The announcement of the BBC's new policy follows pressure from the Food Commission and Parents Jury, prompted by a Tweenies Happy Meals promotion in McDonald's. Many members of the Parents Jury wrote to BBC Worldwide to express their anger at BBC Tweenies characters being used to promote unhealthy food to toddlers.

The *Food Magazine* followed up the story last July by exposing all the other unhealthy products that the BBC was allowing Tweenies to promote.

As a result, BBC Worldwide agreed to meet with the Food Commission, to discuss the development of a BBC nutrition policy.

The Food Commission first challenged BBC Worldwide when we found its Tweenies characters being used to promote high salt, high saturated fat and high sugar McDonald's Happy Meal.

Embarrassed by the media attention that the BBC's announcement stirred up this March, Bob the Builder's agents (HIT Entertainment) contacted the Food Commission. The agents assured us they will be negotiating with Heinz and HP to reduce salt in children's pasta shapes on which Bob the Builder and Thomas the Tank Engine appear.

They have also agreed to meet with the Food Commission and Parents Jury to discuss details of the BBC's nutrition initiative.

Other companies owning the licence to familiar characters have also been in touch, and the Food

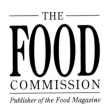

THE
FOOD
COMMISSION
Publisher of the Food Magazine

Commission is planning a round-table meeting to bring these companies together to discuss their responsibilities in promoting food to children.

In summary, BBC Worldwide's new policy stipulates that:

- There will be no more fast food deals for BBC children's characters – nationally and internationally.
- There will be no more 'everyday treat' foods branded with BBC characters, e.g. confectionery, lollies and crisps. BBC Worldwide will continue to allow its children's characters on 'occasional treat foods for special occasions', e.g. Easter eggs.
- Foods carrying BBC characters will conform to salt, fat and sugar guidelines drawn up in partnership with the Food Standards Agency.
- The BBC will seek to use its children's characters to promote healthy staple foods, supporting foods from the major food groups.
- Additive use (e.g. colourings and preservatives) will be reviewed, with the aim of excluding those that may be linked to hyperactivity, asthma or unhealthy reactions.
- Foods carrying BBC children's characters will have clearer and

---

There will be no more 'everyday treat' foods branded with BBC characters, e.g. confectionery, lollies and crisps

---

less misleading labelling. BBC Worldwide research with over 1,000 parents found that they were unhappy with being given the impression that a food was healthy from information on the front of the label, only to find that the ingredients list revealed unhealthy levels of sugar or fat.

The nutritional standards will be communicated to BBC agents worldwide, with final sign-off of any food deals managed by the Director of Children's Operations.

The Food Commission is delighted that the BBC, with its public-service role, has understood what an important part it has to play in improving children's diets. We hope that the agents for other characters will follow suit, and we will contact them over the coming weeks.

These will include companies such as Disney, HIT Entertainment, Warner Bros and Mattel, whose internationally recognised characters include Winnie the Pooh, Bob the Builder, Thomas the Tank Engine, Tom & Jerry and Barbie – all firm favourites with young children.

There are still plenty of products promoted by other children's characters that would be unlikely to comply with the BBC's new nutrition policy.

The BBC's announcement of a nutrition policy has shown, once again, that Parent Power really works. When we sent out news to the Parents Jury, we received many comments in response, typified by this from a Parents Jury member: 'It was good to hear that the parts we played all helped achieve this. Fantastic – and a big thank you to the Food Commission for pulling all the parent power together!'

- The above information is from the Food Commission's website which can be found at www.foodcomm.org.uk

© *The Food Commission*

CHAPTER TWO: FOOD SAFETY

Understanding the food label

By Kate Arthur RD

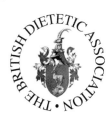

The nutrition panel on the label of most foods and drinks can provide useful information about their nutrition content. Amounts are given per 100g of food and may also be provided per serving of the product, so you can work out how much energy, protein, fat and sugar you will be getting. Some labels give even more information, for example different types of fat, dietary fibre and sodium.

Nutrition information panel
Nutritional information

Typical values (cooked as per instructions)

	Per Flan	Per 100g
Energy	1462 kJ	975 kJ
	351 kcal	234 kcal
Protein	9.0g	6.0g
Carbohydrate	28.2g	18.8g
Of which sugars	3.0g	2.0g
Of which starch	25.2g	16.8g
Fat	22.3g	14.0g
Of which saturates	7.6g	5.1g
Of which monounsaturates	10.9g	7.3g
Of which polyunsaturates	2.7g	1.8g
Fibre	1.6g	1.1g
Sodium	0.6g	0.4g
Per flan	**351 kcal**	**22.3g fat**

Guideline daily amounts
Guideline daily amount

Each day	Women	Men
Calories	2000	2500
Fat	70g	95g
Salt	5g	7g

Official Government figures for average adults

What does the nutrition information mean?
Energy: can be expressed as kJ (kilojoules) or as kcal (kilocalories). Strictly speaking, a kilocalorie is equivalent to 1000 calories, but in everyday language, the term 'calorie' tends to be used for both measures.

Carbohydrate: includes both sugars and starches. The figure given for sugars includes both added sugar and natural sugar (e.g. fruit sugar).

Fat: There are 3 main types of fats listed on food labels: saturates, polyunsaturates and monounsaturates. The label will show the total amount of fat, and may provide information on the different types as well.

Health claims: what do they mean?
To help you choose lower fat and lower sugar options more easily, look for the nutrition claims such as:
- Low fat – indicates the food contains less than 3g fat per 100g/100ml of the food.
- Reduced fat – the food must contain 25% less fat than a similar standard product, it does not mean the product is 'low fat'.

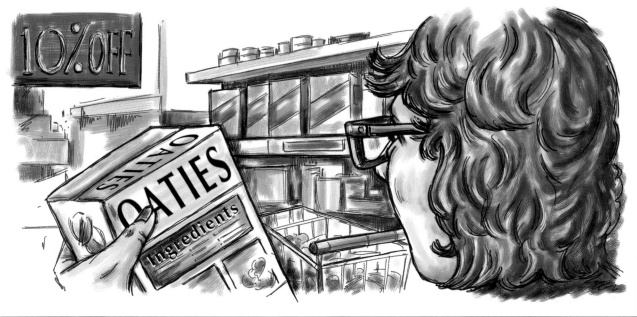

- Less than 5% fat (or 95% fat free) – indicates the food contains less than 5g fat per 100g, for example if you bought a ready meal which had this claim and the serving size was 400g then the whole meal would contain 20g fat. Use these claims as a guide and always check the nutrition panel for the total amount of fat in a serving and compare this with the guideline daily amount.
- X% less fat than the standard product – shows the fat reduction made to a product compared to a standard named product e.g. 20% less fat than a comparable product. This type of claim can

There are 3 main types of fats listed on food labels; saturates, polyunsaturates and mono-unsaturates

help you choose lower fat options, however, always check to see how much fat the product contributes to your guideline daily amount – it may still be high in fat.
- No added sugar – no sugars from any source have been added. May still contain a lot of natural sugar e.g. fruit sugar in fruit juice.

- Low sugar – contains no more than 5g of sugar per 100g / 100ml of food.
- Reduced sugar – must contain 25% less sugar than the regular product.

■ This Food Fact information is a public service of the British Dietetic Association intended for information only. It is not a substitute for proper medical diagnosis or dietary advice given by a Registered Dietitian (RD). To check that your dietitian is Registered check www.hpc-uk.org Other Food Fact sheets are available from www.bda.uk.com

© *The British Dietetic Association*

What do labels tell me?

Labels are there to tell you what you are buying. The law says that the name of a product must not be misleading. Saying 'pâté' isn't enough because there are many kinds – so the label must say what sort of pâté it is. It also has to tell us if the food has undergone a process, such as *UHT* milk, *smoked* mackerel, or *dried* apricots

What should I look for on labels?

Value for money
As well as comparing pack weights, you can use the ingredient list to choose which product you want from the points of view of health, taste and cost.

Remember, the ingredients are listed in descending order of weight.

Freedom of choice
Labels allow you to buy things you like or avoid things you shouldn't eat.

Healthy eating
Most products now label the amount of calories, fat, sugars, fibre and sodium/salt in them.

Remember to act on the information which food labels contain.

What specific nutritional information appears on labels?

Energy
This is the amount of energy – calories – that the food will give you when you eat it. It is measured either in calories (kcal) or joules (kJ).

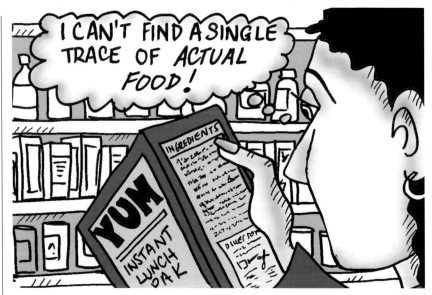

Protein
Protein is important for body growth and repair. Most adults get more than enough protein for their needs.

Carbohydrate
Mainly sugars and starch. Most labels tell you how much of the total carbohydrate is sugars (the remainder is mostly starch).

Starch
We should get most of our energy from starch, rather than from fats

and sugars. (Foods with plenty of starch include bread, breakfast cereals, rice, pasta and potatoes.)

Sugars
This covers both sugars which occur naturally in fruit and milk, and added sugar. Added sugars can cause tooth decay when eaten frequently.

Saturated fat
This type of fat may raise blood cholesterol levels, which can cause heart disease. (For a healthy heart,

cut back on saturates, for example, pies, sausages, butter, cheese, cakes and biscuits.)

Monounsaturated and polyunsaturated fat

Monounsaturates are neutral for heart disease, and polyunsaturates lower blood cholesterol levels. It is better to eat foods rich in monounsaturates (olive oil and rapeseed oil) and polyunsaturates (sunflower oil and soya oil), than foods rich in saturates.

But remember, they are still fats.

Dietary fibre

Fibre helps prevent constipation, piles and bowel problems. (Good sources of fibre are baked beans, kidney beans, high-fibre breakfast cereals, wholemeal bread, fruit and vegetables.)

Sodium

Most sodium in food is from salt. Sodium can help to cause high blood pressure. More than two-thirds of the sodium we eat comes from processed foods, so check the nutrition label to cut back on it.

Can labels say what they like?

No. Food labelling is strictly governed by law. A food can't claim to be 'reduced calorie' unless it is much lower in calories than the usual version. However, you should be aware of certain claims.

You should treat claims like 'low-fat', 'reduced-sodium' and 'high-fibre' with care. Although by law these claims should not be mis-

---

Food labelling is strictly governed by law. A food can't claim to be 'reduced calorie' unless it is much lower in calories than the usual version

---

leading, there are no legal definitions for quantities (except for butter, margarine and other spreadable fats).

And don't forget that with sugar, the way you eat the food is as important as the amount of sugar it contains. Claims like 'low sugar' and 'reduced sugar' are only important on foods and drinks such as sweets, biscuits and soft drinks.

Are there any rules about pictures on labels?

Food packaging pictures must not mislead.

A raspberry yogurt that gets its flavour from artificial flavouring, and not from fruit, cannot have a picture of raspberries on the pot.

What about descriptions of things on labels?

A few well-known foods are allowed to keep their names because we know what they are.

After all, we know that cream crackers don't contain cream, and that Swiss rolls don't have to come from Switzerland.

But if something we expect to come from one place – such as Cornish

---

clotted cream – isn't made there, the label must state where it is made.

Are labelling ingredients listed in any particular order?

Yes. All ingredients, including additives, are listed in descending order of weight at the time they were used to make the food. If flavourings are used, the packet must say so.

As well as this information, there will also be the manufacturer's name and address, a datemark, instructions for safe storage and an indicated weight.

Should I heed all label advice?

Yes, paying particular attention to:
- Date instructions, such as 'Use by' and 'Best before', to avoid or reduce the risk of food poisoning.
- Defrosting and cooking times (to ensure that any harmful bugs are killed).
- Storage instructions and directions for preparing food (as correct handling can protect us against illness).

Don't worry if the 'Display until' date has been reached. These are instructions to shop staff rather than us. Just check the 'Use by' or 'Best before' date stamps instead.

And remember, don't eat or cook anything about which you are unsure. If in doubt – throw it out.

■ The above information is from the Government's Food Standards Agency's website which can be found at www.foodstandards.gov.uk

© Crown copyright

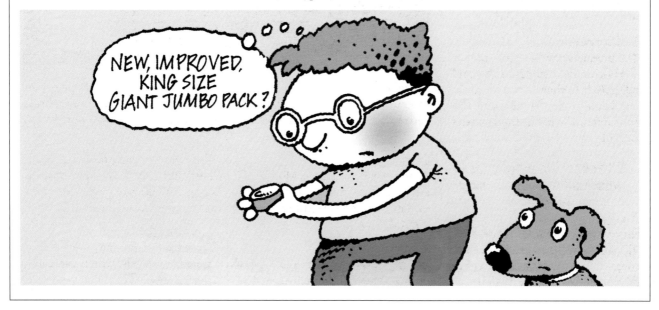

Reading between the lines

It looks like there's a long way to go before it becomes a legal requirement to provide honest and clear food labelling that helps people to opt for a healthy diet

By Daloni Carlisle

Every day, in every one of its shops, the Co-op is breaking the law by using detailed labels that tell shoppers what's in the food they are buying. It describes, for example, whether a food has a 'high', 'medium' or 'low' fat content and it gives the salt content in milligrams. Dr Cath Humphries, its chief scientific adviser, doesn't expect to end up in court, though. 'We are very friendly with our enforcement people. They understand we have consumers' best interests at heart – and we are not misleading anyone.' The Co-op's customers feel the same way. In opinion polls, they consistently praise its brave stand in providing meaningful labels.

The battle for better labelling is not new. But the Consumers' Association (CA), which has been campaigning for honest information for several years, believes labels matter more now than ever before. 'Consumers are increasingly reliant on labels,' says senior public affairs officer, Peter Jenkins. 'We shop in a hurry. We shop more at supermarkets. We eat more processed food and food production is becoming more complex.' Consumers aiming for a healthy diet also rely on labels to turn nutrition advice into reality.

The Co-op's food labels can be traced back to 1997 and its report, *Lie of the Label*, published in conjunction with Sustain – the alliance for food and better farming – and the CA. The report highlighted how food retailers and manufacturers misled the public into thinking the food they were buying was better than it actually was – largely through what the report called the 'seven deadly sins' (see box). In response, the Co-op put forward a code of practice for honest labelling, which now forms the basis of its own labels – and urged the rest of the food industry to follow suit. But despite a flurry of initiatives, a second report (published in 2002) found that labels still mislead consumers – and the law still offers little protection. 'Particularly alarming is the lack of progress on nutrition labelling,' says *Lie of the Label II*. That's despite the fact that, 'There has been a series of warnings by food and health experts that our diet is contributing to a growth in obesity and other health problems in the UK, including among children.'

Humphries says it is not just the misleading claims that are to blame for poor information. The regulatory framework must also share responsibility. 'Basically it was evolved by nutritionists who see the whole thing from a scientific viewpoint,' she says. 'So while it makes scientific sense if you have learned about energy and carbohydrate and fat, it is not much use otherwise.' Jeanette Longfield, Sustain's coordinator, agrees. She also describes the law – which makes nutrition labelling voluntary – as 'deeply flawed'.

EC law, enacted in this country through the Food Labelling Regulations 1996 (as amended), offers two formats for nutrition labels – although there is no compulsion to use either unless a nutrition claim is made. Manufacturers can list either the 'Big Four' nutrients (energy, protein, carbohydrate and fat) or the 'Full Eight' (the Big Four plus sugars, saturates, fibre and sodium). *Lie of the Label II* cites research showing that a quarter of people do not know that sugar and carbohydrate are related (it's only when manufacturers opt for the Full Eight that both are listed). Again, the law says only sodium may be listed – but most shoppers don't relate sodium to salt (and very few know that you need to multiply the sodium content by two and a half to get a rough idea of the amount of salt present).

Alcohol labelling is another area of concern, according to Humphries. 'Legally you are not allowed to list ingredients, the units of alcohol in a serving, the amount of calories or put sensible drinking advice.' Again, the Co-op provides all this information. So what hope is there for change?

The Food and Drink Federation (FDF) rejects the findings of *Lie of the Label II*, saying: 'Industry agrees that marketing claims and labelling should be truthful and not misleading. The 1990 Food Safety Act protects consumers from claims that fail these tests.' The FDF is working with the Food Standards Agency (FSA) on its Food Labelling Action

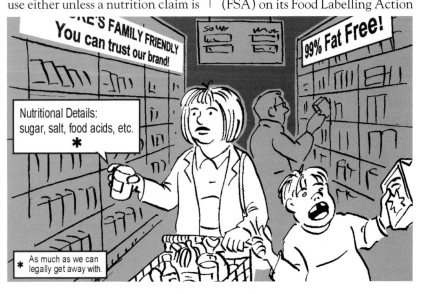

The Seven Deadly Sins

1. **The Illusion:** Labels that hide information. It might say, for instance, 'mince and onion' when the main ingredient is actually mechanically recovered chicken.
2. **Weasel Words:** Labels that use nice words that don't mean very much, such as 'natural', 'wholesome' or 'traditional'.
3. **Rose-tinted Spectacles:** Where pictures on the pack make the food look better than what's actually on offer inside.
4. **The Bluff:** Making the food sound special because it's free of something. For example, dried pasta labelled 'free from preservatives' when, by law, it's not allowed any preservatives.
5. **The Hidden Truth:** Crucial information is hidden away where it can't easily be seen. For instance, the minimum percentage meat content.
6. **The Half Truth:** Labels that tell you what isn't in the product. For example, '80% fat free' actually means 20% of the produce is fat (way above the 3% allowed for a 'low fat' claim).
7. **Small Print:** Where you need a magnifying glass to read all but the hard sell on the front.

Source: *Lie of the Label*

The Parents Jury

Twelve parents, angry at the way food is marketed to their children, formed the Parents Jury at the Food Commission in March 2002. By the end of the year, more than 1,000 parents had joined.

According to research officer Kath Dalmeny, the marketing methods used by companies make it really difficult for parents to ensure their children have a healthy diet. Parents, she says, are pitched against Teletubby puddings, David Beckham promoting Pepsi and packaging designed for 'mum appeal' – with messages about vitamins and minerals belying the high sugar and salt content within products.

The Parents Jury will shortly announce the winners of the 2003 awards for the labelling of children's food. It will award good practice, as well as looking at 'label fibs' – the products claiming to be rich in calcium in big letters, while hiding a high sugar content in the small print. A 'food heroes' and 'greedy stars' category will name pop stars and footballers who endorse either healthy or unhealthy products.

Name and Shame

The Consumers' Association is campaigning for better labelling, in particular it wants: labelling of GM derivatives; full nutrition details on pre-packed foods; and a full list of ingredients on all food products.

The campaign has two prongs: lobbying at European Commission and government level; and a 'name and shame' initiative, in which it investigates complaints from members and then goes on to try and force manufacturers to make a change.

Successes so far include:
- Marks and Spencer agreed to withdraw a 'Count on us . . .' barbecue marinade which the Consumers Association revealed was higher in calories than its standard equivalent.
- United Foods International agreed to change the label on its Grove Fresh Cranberry and Apple Juice to Apple and Cranberry as it contains only 7.5% cranberry juice.
- Yeo Valley is replacing the word 'healthy' on packets of Organic Creme Fraiche with 'healthier', which more accurately describes a product containing 17.5% fat.

Plan, an ongoing programme of work set up in 2000 and involving industry and consumer groups.

The FSA, which has a remit 'to help people to eat more healthily', points to a raft of initiatives already resulting from this plan. For example, in 2002 it published advice on the use of terms such as 'fresh' and 'natural'. Currently, it is consulting on rules to tackle the mislabelling of chicken breast fillets that contain added water, beef or pork proteins. In addition, new formats for nutrition labels are being tested. The problem is, the food industry is not compelled to take FSA advice that isn't backed by EC law.

On the plus side, the EC is reviewing labelling law – and new directives are being issued on a monthly basis. Rules to define 'meat' have been agreed, for example, along with new directives on listing potential allergens and caffeine content (the latter is an issue of particular concern to pregnant women who need to keep caffeine levels low). There are even new proposals for regulating nutrition and health claims – a move that's welcomed by the Consumers' Association. Nevertheless, Jeanette Longfield at Sustain says that the pace of change at the EC is 'glacial' – and she feels that the industry 'is twiddling its thumbs'.

In the UK, small victories are being won every week through the Food Commission's Parents Jury (see second box) and the CA's 'name and shame' campaign (see third box). Overall, however, the chances of getting useful, easy-to-understand labels into general circulation – certainly in the short term – remains bleak. 'As consumers, I think the only thing we can do is be extremely sceptical about what's in front of our eyes,' says Longfield. 'If you're interested in key ingredients because of a medical condition, or for healthy eating, you are going to have to learn to do sums and carry a calculator.'

■ The above information is from the magazine *Health Development Today* published by the Health Development Agency. Visit their website at www.hda.nhs.uk

© *Health Development Agency*

Consumer attitudes towards food

Information from the Food Standards Agency

The Food Standards Agency has published its fourth UK-wide *Consumer Attitudes to Food Survey* which provides the Agency with information covering consumer attitudes, knowledge, behaviour and awareness of food issues.

The survey was devised to help track any changes in consumer opinions about food, since the Agency was set up in April 2000. This helps the Agency improve its knowledge and understanding of consumer views; as well as to help gauge changes of public confidence in food safety.

The 2003 survey highlights a number of key trends that have emerged since 2000, these include:

- A significant decline in consumer concern over BSE (down to 42% in 2003 from 61% in 2000)
- A decline in consumer concern about the safety of meat – particularly raw meat (down to 63% in 2003 from 70% in 2000) and raw beef (down to 38% in 2003 from 53% in 2000)
- A decline in consumer concern over eggs (down to 20% in 2003 from 26% in 2000)
- A year-on-year increase in the number of consumers who are aware that we should eat 5 portions of a variety of fruit and veg each day (up from 43% in 2000 to 59% in 2003). In terms of social class, 76% of the ABs were aware that we should eat 'at least 5 portions per day', falling to 61% among the C1C2s and down to 41% among DEs.
- Significant rise in the number of consumers that look for the total salt content in a product by checking the nutritional information on food labels. This was up from 22% in 2000 to 36% in 2003
- One-third of consumers (37%) felt that they had changed their eating habits over the last year and were now eating more healthily, with only 6% believing that their diet was currently less healthy than a year ago.

Summary of other findings:

Food labelling

- 78% of consumers claim to check food labels, 31% always, 26% usually and 21% occasionally
- 60% of consumers found information on food labelling easy to understand. However, one in five consumers found some food labels 'fairly difficult' to understand, and one in twenty found them 'very difficult'
- Two-fifths of consumers are concerned about the accuracy of food labelling compared to around a third in previous years
- Just over half (52%) of UK consumers are concerned about the accuracy of health claims, although the majority of concerned consumers (58%) were 'fairly' rather than 'very concerned'.

Food safety

- Year-on-year decrease in the number of consumers that feel that food safety is 'a lot' worse (6% in 2000, 5% in 2001, 4% in 2002, 4% in 2003)
- Level of concern about GM foods remains similar to the past two years (38% of consumers expressed concern in 2003, compared to 43% in 2000)
- Significant increase in the number of consumers who expressed concern over ready-made meals, up to 17% in 2003 from 13% in 2002
- Half of the consumers interviewed were concerned about the amount of fat (53%), salt (50%) and sugar (47%) in food, with these concerns affecting claimed eating habits.

Food-borne disease

- Between a third and a half of all consumers surveyed claimed to change their eating habits in 2003 as a result of increased concern over hygiene in catering establishments – with 70% no longer buying food from an outlet where they had concerns about hygiene
- An increase in the number of consumers who believe they may have experienced a bout of diarrhoea/vomiting in the last 12 months. 16% in 2003, compared with 13% in both 2000 and 2002
- A year-on-year increase in consumer concern about hygiene in mobile food outlets (from 26% in 2002 up to 30% in 2003).

Key differences across groups

- Women are more likely to be aware of food issues and more concerned about food safety
- People between the ages of 16-25 and over 66 tend to be less knowledgeable and less concerned about food issues.

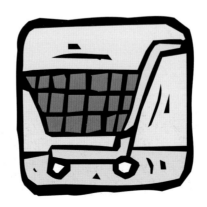

- The above information is an extract from the summary of the Food Standards Agency's report *Consumer Attitudes to Food Survey 2004*. For further information visit their website at www.food.gov.uk

Food poisoning

Information from the Food and Drink Federation

Each year it is estimated that as many as 5.5 million people in the UK may suffer from food-borne illnesses – that's 1 in 10 people. This article explains what food poisoning is and describes some of the most common germs that cause it.

More information on this can be found from the Food Standards Agency website – www.food.gov.uk

About germs

Germs are invisible except under a powerful microscope; hence the name micro-organisms or microbes. Microbes can be grouped according to their different structures; two common groups of microbes are viruses and bacteria. Not all bacteria are harmful – indeed many are essential for life. The bacteria, viruses and other microbes that cause illness are commonly known as germs.

Germs found in food can lead to food poisoning which can be dangerous and can kill – though this is rare. They are very hard to detect since they do not usually affect the taste, appearance or smell of food.

The most serious types of food poisoning are due to bacteria. The more bacteria present, the more likely you are to become ill. Bacteria multiply fast and to do so need moisture, food, warmth and time. The presence or absence of oxygen, salt, sugar and the acidity of the

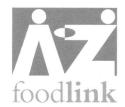

surroundings are also important factors. In the right conditions one bacterium can multiply to more than 4 million in just 8 hours.

They multiply best between 5 and 63°C but are killed at temperatures of 70°C. At temperatures below 5°C, most bacteria multiply very slowly, if at all. At very low temperatures some bacteria will die, but many survive and can start to multiply again if warm conditions return. That is why proper cooking and chilling of food can help reduce the risk of food poisoning.

Food poisoning

Germs can get into our food at any point in the food chain – from the time when an animal or food is in the field to the moment food is put on to the table to eat.

If they are allowed to survive and multiply, they can cause illness when that food is eaten.

Sometimes these germs are spread to other foods, for example via hands or kitchen utensils, and cause illness when those foods are eaten. This is known as cross-contamination.

The symptoms of food poisoning can last for days and include abdominal pains, diarrhoea, vomiting, nausea and fever. The symptoms usually come on suddenly, but can occur several days after eating contaminated food. They will usually get better on their own. Your pharmacist may be able to advise on suitable remedies or contact NHS Direct. If symptoms persist contact your doctor. Symptoms such as diarrhoea and vomiting are not always due to food poisoning but if you think you have food poisoning contact your local Environmental Health Officer.

Food poisoning outbreaks

Sometimes groups of people can be infected at the same time. They may have eaten at a party, or restaurant, or there may be a batch of contaminated food being sold in different places. In such cases Environmental Health Officers (EHOs), who are employed by Local Authorities, will usually investigate the matter to find out the cause. EHOs will alert others to the dangers, offer advice, and where necessary prosecute offenders for breaches of food safety laws. Whenever such outbreaks of food poisoning occur or are suspected, it is important to contact an EHO; they can be found in the local council section of the phone book.

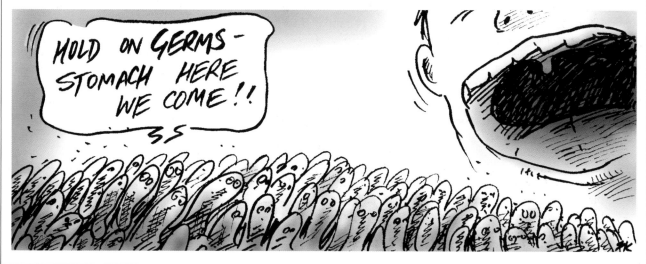

Seeking advice

EHOs are also happy to provide advice on food safety to local businesses. Another source of advice is the Food Standards Agency, their website address is www.food.gov.uk

Vulnerable groups

Food poisoning is more likely to affect people with lowered resistance to disease than healthy people who might show mild symptoms or none at all. Elderly or sick people, babies, young children and pregnant women are particularly vulnerable to food poisoning. Seek treatment if they have symptoms. Extra care should also be taken when preparing food for, and looking after, these vulnerable groups to minimise the risks of their coming into contact with food poisoning bacteria.

Avoiding food poisoning

Most food poisoning is preventable although it isn't possible to completely eliminate the risk. For further advice see our other Fact Files on Food Storage, Food Hygiene and Food Preparation.

More about microbes

Here is some more information about the most common microbes that cause food poisoning. More information on this can be found from the Food Standards Agency website – www.food.gov.uk

Campylobacter

Source

Campylobacter can be found in raw poultry and meat, unpasteurised milk, and untreated water. Pasteurised milk can be contaminated by birds pecking bottle tops on the doorstep. Pets with diarrhoea can also be a source of infection. Campylobacter is the most common identified cause of food poisoning.

Characteristics

Illness may be caused by a small number of bacteria. Cross-contamination can lead to illness. Thorough cooking and pasteurisation of milk will destroy Campylobacter.

Symptoms

Symptoms include fever, headache and a feeling of being unwell, followed by severe abdominal pain

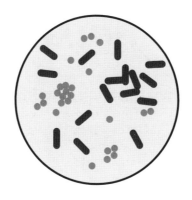

and diarrhoea which may be bloody. Symptoms normally take 2-5 days to appear but it can be as long as 10 days and return over a number of weeks.

Salmonella

Source

Salmonella has been found in raw meat, poultry and eggs, raw unwashed vegetables, unpasteurised milk and dairy products and many other types of food. It is found in the gut and faeces of animals and humans. Salmonella is the second most common cause of food poisoning.

Characteristics

Salmonella survives when refrigerated although it is unable to multiply through cooking and pasteurisation. Usually large numbers of the bacteria are needed to cause infection but outbreaks have been reported where infection has been caused by a low number of bacteria.

Symptoms

It normally takes 12 to 48 hours for symptoms to develop. Symptoms may include fever, diarrhoea, vomiting and abdominal pain. Infection may be very severe, and in some cases may be fatal. It is particularly likely to cause severe illness in the very young and very old. Symptoms may last up to three weeks and there may be complications such as reactive arthritis.

E. COLI

Source

E. coli is a widespread organism that is normally found in the guts of animals and humans. There are many different types, some of which are capable of causing illness. One uncommon type which can cause serious illness is Verocytotoxin producing E. coli O157 which has been found in raw and undercooked

meats, unpasteurised milk and dairy products, raw vegetables and unpasteurised apple juice.

Characteristics

Illness may be caused by a small number of bacteria, so cross-contamination can lead to illness. The bacteria can survive refrigeration and freezer storage, but thorough cooking of food and pasteurisation of milk will kill them.

Symptoms

Symptoms normally take about 2 days to develop but may start within a day, or take up to 5 days to come on. The main symptom is diarrhoea. In some cases, particularly in children under the age of 6 and in the elderly, infection can lead to diarrhoea which may be bloody and severe, kidney failure, and sometimes death.

Clostridium perfringens

Source

Clostridium perfringens is excreted by a wide range of animals. It can be found in soil, animal manure, and sewage, and also in raw meat and poultry.

Characteristics

Clostridium perfringens produces spores which may not be killed during cooking. If foods are allowed to cool slowly, the spores germinate and produce bacteria which grow rapidly. These bacteria may not be killed if the food is not reheated until it is piping hot. It is particularly associated with gravies, cooked meat dishes, stews and pies and very large joints of meat and poultry.

Symptoms

Symptoms are mainly abdominal pain, diarrhoea and sometimes nausea starting usually 8-18 hours after eating the food. It may be fatal in the elderly and debilitated.

Listeria

Source

Listeria is widely present in the environment. It is found in soil, vegetation, raw milk, meat, poultry, cheeses (particularly soft mould-ripened varieties) and salad vegetables. It is also found in the guts of animals and humans. One type, Listeria monocytogenes, can cause illness in humans.

Characteristics

Listeria monocytogenes, unlike most other food poisoning bacteria, can grow at low temperatures, even in the fridge. Thorough cooking of food and pasteurisation of milk will destroy Listeria.

Symptoms

It can take days or weeks for symptoms to develop. Symptoms can range from mild flu-like illness to meningitis and septicaemia; and in pregnant women, abortion, miscarriage or birth of an infected child. Other susceptible groups are those whose immune systems are compromised, the very young and the very old. People in these groups are advised to avoid certain foods, such as soft mould-ripened cheeses and pâtés, because of the risk of severe infection.

Bacillus cereus

Source

Bacillus cereus is found in soil and dust. It is frequently found in rice dishes, occasionally pasta, meat or vegetable dishes, dairy products, soups, sauces and sweet pastry products where these have not been cooled quickly and effectively after cooking and during storage.

Characteristics

Illness may be caused by a small number of bacteria, so cross-contamination can lead to illness. The bacteria can form spores; they are not easily destroyed by heat and will survive cooking of food. If food is cooled slowly or kept warm for some time before serving, the spores will germinate and produce bacteria. Bacteria can multiply rapidly at these temperatures and produce a very heat-resistant toxin which will not be destroyed by subsequent reheating.

Symptoms

Bacillus cereus can cause two distinct types of illness – a diarrhoeal form (diarrhoea and abdominal pain) with an incubation period of 8 to 16 hours and an emetic form (primarily vomiting, possibly with diarrhoea) with an incubation period of 1 to 5 hours. In both types the illness usually lasts less than 24 hours after onset.

Staphylococcus aureus

Source

Staphylococcus aureus may be found on the skin, in infected cuts and boils and in the nose. It may also be found in unpasteurised milk. It can be transferred to food from the hands or from droplets from the nose or mouth.

Characteristics

Food poisoning from Staphylococcus aureus follows the consumption of heavily contaminated food, where bacteria have multiplied and produced a toxin which causes illness when the food is consumed. Staphylococcus aureus survives when refrigerated although it does not multiply. The bacteria are destroyed by pasteurisation of milk and cooking of food, but the toxin may survive these processes. The main foods associated with illness are cooked meats, poultry and foods which are handled during preparation without subsequent cooking.

Symptoms

Onset of symptoms varies between 2 and 6 hours. Symptoms are severe vomiting, abdominal pains and diarrhoea. They generally last no longer than 2 days.

Norwalk-like viruses

(Previously know as Small Round Structured Viruses or SRSVs)

Source

Norwalk-like viruses are the commonest food-borne viral infection and are usually spread from person to person.

Characteristics

Norwalk-like viruses are transmitted from person to person (e.g. by projectile vomiting), environmental contamination and contaminated water. Food-borne infection may be associated with sewage contamination of shellfish or fresh produce, or contamination by an infected food handler. Outbreaks occur most frequently in nursing homes and hospitals due to person-to-person spread.

Symptoms

Norwalk-like viruses cause an acute gastro-enteritis and are the commonest cause of viral gastro-enteritis epidemics. Symptoms include vomiting and diarrhoea. The symptoms take 12-48 hours to develop, and last for about 2 days.

■ The above information is from the Food and Drink Federation's foodlink website which can be found at www.foodlink.org.uk

© Food and Drink Federation

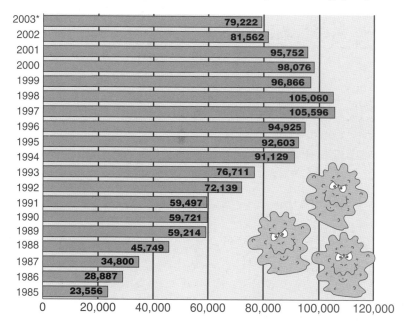

Food poisoning statistics

Number of notified cases of food poisoning (UK)

2003*	79,222
2002	81,562
2001	95,752
2000	98,076
1999	96,866
1998	105,060
1997	105,596
1996	94,925
1995	92,603
1994	91,129
1993	76,711
1992	72,139
1991	59,497
1990	59,721
1989	59,214
1988	45,749
1987	34,800
1986	28,887
1985	23,556

Source: Office of Population Censuses and Surveys, Scottish Centre for Infection and Environmental Health and Regional Information Branch, Department of Health and Social Security, Belfast
* denotes provisional figures.

Source: foodlink, Food and Drink Federation

Healthy eating branded 'illegal'

Supermarkets are being prosecuted for telling shoppers that fruit and vegetables are good for them.

Tesco is being taken to court for running a promotion in partnership with a leading charity encouraging people to eat healthily in a bid to prevent cancer. Asda faces a similar prosecution.

The bizarre red-tape prosecutions are being brought by trading standards departments from two different local councils, which claim the stores have flouted laws governing labelling and health claims.

Tesco, in association with Cancer Research UK, printed labels on millions of pre-packed fruit and vegetables advising: 'Eat at least 5 different portions of fruit and veg a day to help prevent cancer.'

Cancer prevention

Asda's prosecution surrounds marketing material stating: 'Mangoes are a great source of vitamin C and beta-carotene, which are good for healthy eyes and skin. Their anti-oxidant properties help to fight cancer.'

No one is disputing that these claims are true. However, it appears that it is illegal to apply them to a particular product.

Trading standards officers claim the supermarkets are in breach of the 1939 Cancer Act, which was brought in to stop people selling quack cures, and the 1996 Food Labelling regulations.

Tesco, which is being prosecuted by Shropshire County Council, has been forced to water down the health message on its labels. However, the council will continue with the prosecution next month at West Mercia Magistrates' Court.

No one is disputing that these claims are true. However, it appears that it is illegal to apply them to a particular product

---

The store's marketing director, Tim Mason, said: 'It is crazy that we are being prosecuted for promoting a responsible health message.'

Asda, which is being prosecuted by Swindon council, said: 'We are disappointed that the local authority is continuing to pursue the matter, given that we have sought to follow one of the Government's policy objectives.'

Food regulations

A spokesman for Swindon council said: 'Our view is that there is a clear breach of both the Cancer Act and Food Labelling regulations. You cannot make health claims suggesting a product will prevent cancer.'

The stores could be fined £1,000 for each breach of the Cancer Act and £5,000 for each offence under the Food Labelling regulations.

Cancer Research UK said it was 'very disappointed' by the Tesco prosecution. And the British Retail Consortium has written to Public Health Minister Melanie Johnson pointing out the folly of the prosecutions.

The Government claimed in a 2000 NHS Plan that 'increasing fruit and vegetable consumption is the second most effective strategy to reduce the risk of cancer'.

■ This article first appeared in the *Daily Mail*, May 2004.

© 2004 Associated Newspapers Ltd

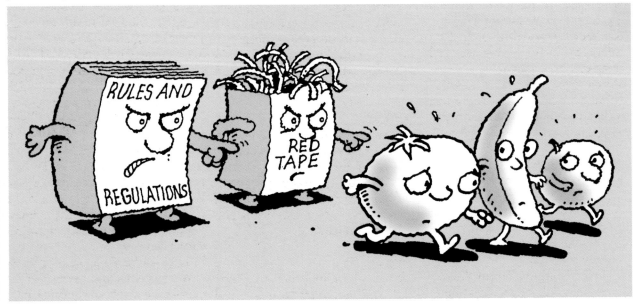

Food and farming

Information from Friends of the Earth

Food matters

Wherever you live and whatever you earn, food is essential for life. But what we eat, how it is produced and where we buy it are complicated issues in 21st-century Britain.

Today very few of us are involved in growing our own food or raising animals, and we buy over 75 per cent of our food from supermarkets. But we worry, more than ever, about the safety of the food we buy and the possible toxins we and our children might be eating.

Farming is now in crisis, and many rural communities are declining. Many smaller farmers, forced to produce at the lowest possible cost because of pressure from supermarkets, can no longer make a living from growing food. Cheap food is imported from hundreds or even thousands of miles away, burning up fuel which is adding to dangerous climate change.

Intensive farming in this country continues to damage the environment and put profit above people, wildlife and animal welfare. And the global system for governing food policy is making the corporations rich while farmers in developing countries can no longer afford to feed their families.

That's why Friends of the Earth is campaigning for sustainable and equitable food production for everyone. We can provide high quality food without trashing the environment and threatening our wildlife. This article shows how sustainable ways of farming can provide a decent living for farmers and give us safe, nutritious food, at a price we can afford.

Did you know?

- In 1939 there were half a million farms in the UK employing 15 per cent of the population. In 2000 only two per cent of the population still worked in agriculture.
- In 2002 the Environment Agency estimated that intensive farming

Friends of the Earth

costs the country £500 million each year because of water pollution, soil erosion and resulting flood damage.

- The average distance food has travelled from field to plate (food miles) has doubled in the past 20 years.
- On average, only 10 pence in every pound spent in a supermarket goes to the person who actually grew the food.

What's in your shopping bag?

Fruit and vegetables

Many, especially those that are out of season, are imported from thousands of miles away by aircraft, burning fuel and adding to climate change. Over 50 per cent may also have pesticide residues in them. Yet we could support sustainable farming by buying local and organic food.

Processed food

Highly processed food typically contains high levels of salt, sugar and fats. Excessive consumption is adding to obesity problems for people in the UK. The National Audit Office says the cost of obesity is £2.5 billion a year.

Chicken

Almost all poultry in the UK are raised in cramped, unhealthy conditions. If we ate a smaller quantity of high-quality, free-range meat, it would improve animal welfare, save resources, reduce pollution and create farm jobs.

Water

Roughly 1.5 million tonnes of plastic are used every year by the bottled

water industry, creating serious waste problems. Tap water costs about 1000 times less then bottled water, and in most EU countries, including the UK, is actually as good as bottled water.

Bread

New GM labelling regulations allow up to 0.9 per cent of soya flour used in bread to be GM and unlabelled. Supermarkets need to give consumers what they want – GM-free food.

Chocolate

Most cocoa beans used to make chocolate are harvested in Africa where rich countries control the price paid to farmers which is far too low for a decent standard of living. But we could support those farmers by buying chocolate that carries the Fair Trade label. However, chocolate companies should guarantee fair prices to all growers.

Farming in crisis

Over the past 50 years farming has become highly mechanised, dependent on agro-chemicals and very wasteful in its energy use. Such intensive farming creates widespread environmental and health problems.

Pesticides, fertilisers and animal waste pollute our land and water supplies, while destroying and degrading wildlife habitats. Added to this, the food health scares and animal diseases of the past 20 years – e-coli, salmonella, BSE and foot and mouth – are all symptoms of an ailing system which is not sustainable, economically or environmentally.

Intensive farming also receives vast subsidies. Sustainable farming methods and environmental schemes on farms receive far less financial support. And farmers are at the mercy of governments, big businesses and international trade agreements which view farming as a business like any other. The low-cost approach forced on farmers by this system means many simply cannot make a living from growing food.

Supermarkets sell us three-quarters of our food. They have been forcing down prices paid to farmers for years, and can force farmers to sell at or below the cost of production. Their enormous influence over the food business also makes it harder for small shops and small-scale producers to survive.

Intensive farming methods are the product of Government farming policies of the past 50 years. We need a new system that supports farmers who protect wildlife and gives them a fair price for the food they produce. The best way to do this is to support sustainable farming (like organic farming) and localised food production.

Did you know?

- 18,000 jobs in agriculture were lost in 2002 and many small farms went out of business. Some 65,000 people left farming in the six years up to 2002.
- In 2000, 80 per cent of Government subsidies went to intensive production, and only eight per cent went to schemes encouraging farmers to improve the environmental value of the farm.
- Under intensive farming 98 per cent of our wildflower meadows have disappeared, numbers of farmland birds have declined dramatically and our ancient woodlands have been reduced to a fraction of what existed before the war.

Food safety
Genetic modification (GM)
There are natural barriers to stop unrelated species breeding with each other, but advances in biotechnology mean that scientists can now move genetic material from one species to another. But scientists still don't know the full effects of growing GM plants out in the field, where they can cross-pollinate with wild plants and neighbouring crops. They don't know whether introduced genes can cause long-term health effects once they are in the food chain. And they don't know whether genes from crops modified to tolerate weedkillers could transfer into other plants, leading to the development of 'super weeds', resistant to weedkillers.

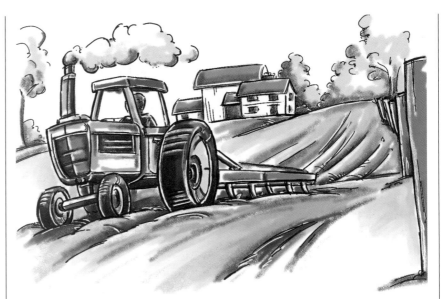

Pesticides
A healthy diet must include fresh fruit and vegetables but Government figures show that half of those sold in supermarkets contain pesticide residues. And we still don't know what the long-term health effects of ingesting a cocktail of pesticide residues are. But we know that the effects on wildlife and the environment can be devastating.

GM technology and pesticides enable intensive agriculture to dominate farming. But sustainable agriculture, locally produced, can provide us with enough to eat, safeguard our wildlife and protect human health.

Did you know?

- Studies in agricultural communities around the world have found links between pesticide exposure and health effects in children, including birth defects.
- A poll in 2001 showed that 70 per cent of Europeans do not want to eat GM food.
- In 2000 the UK Government spent 30 per cent of its food research budget on biotechnology and GM but only eight per cent on organic farming.
- Genetic engineers can put novel genes into any crop. For example, in the laboratory fish genes were put into sweetcorn to make it frost-resistant.

Sustainable farming
Sustainable farming uses non-polluting methods as close as possible to those found in nature. Soil fertility is improved using manure and compost. Artificial fertilisers, pesticides, antibiotics, hormones and GM ingredients are avoided. Reliance on fossil fuels is reduced by cutting out man-made chemicals and reducing food miles. Food production, processing and distribution are carried out as close together as they can be.

Wildlife and conservation
Sustainable farming methods naturally support nature conservation, and reverse the trends in intensive farming which have caused populations of wildlife to decline. Biodiversity (the range and number of wild plants and animals) can be much higher on sustainable farms than intensive farms.

Pesticides
Intensive farmers have 446 artificial pesticides to choose from and they rely on chemical control. Sustainable farming finds ways to avoid using artificial pesticides, such as running mixed farms and encouraging natural predators like ladybirds to keep pest numbers down.

Animal welfare
The production of free-range meat on sustainable farms gives animal welfare high priority. Animals have the space to live in social groups, while GM feed is banned and the use of antibiotics is restricted.

Sustainable, local agriculture is the best way to produce safe, nutritious food which safeguards human health, protects the environment and creates jobs.

- Studies have shown that when an out-of-town supermarket opens, more local jobs are lost than created and many local shops close down.
- If intensive farmers had to pay the costs of cleaning up the environment from pesticides and fertilisers, the price we pay for their food would be higher.
- Organic farms in lowland areas support 40 per cent more birds, double the number of butterflies and 500 per cent more plant species than intensive farms.

What you can do

We can all make choices about what we eat and what we buy that will make a difference.

Buy organic food

Organic farming is one example of sustainable farming. Organic certification means food is produced according to strict rules which have benefits for the environment, our health and animal welfare. Organic food should be free of pesticide residues, antibiotics, hormones or GM ingredients. For these reasons, and if you can afford it, buy organic food. But because 70 per cent of the organic food available is imported it's also worth looking out for local food initiatives.

Buy local food

Eating locally-produced, fresh, seasonal food is good for us and good for the environment. Cutting the number of miles your food has travelled and avoiding packaging reduces pollution and waste. Revitalising local food economies by supporting local producers is the best way to get fresh, healthy food to people on low incomes, and it helps neighbourhood regeneration. If the supermarket is your only option, ask it to stock more locally-produced and more organic foods.

Did you know?

- In 2001 there were 2,500 certified organic producers in the UK, and in 2003 there were 4,100.
- In March 2002 a survey found that food sold at farmers' markets in the South West was on average 35 per cent cheaper than food of similar quality in supermarkets in the same towns.
- In the middle of the UK apple season in 2003 a Friends of the Earth survey found that the majority of apples stocked by Asda and Tesco were imported.

Buy direct from the farmer

Direct links between you and the producer mean the farmer gets a better profit and you can have more confidence that what you buy is produced sustainably. Farmers' markets and farm shops also boost the local rural economy and benefit local farmers. You may be lucky enough to have these nearby, or you can use a delivery scheme which supplies local fruit and vegetables direct to your door (which also cuts packaging waste).

Grow your own

If you have a garden or an allotment, growing food is one of the best ways to guarantee yourself fresh, chemical-free food without clocking up any food miles. Making and using your own compost will cut waste, improve your soil and feed your plants.

Avoid GM foods

Consumers have overwhelmingly rejected GM foods, and supermarkets no longer stock them. From April 2002 all ingredients with a GM content above 0.9 per cent have to be labelled. Some unlabelled foods could contain small amounts of GM and a few products will be labelled – look out for the labelling. Avoid these as much as you can and buy fresh fruit and vegetables and organic foods which are GM-free.

Buy fair trade products

The World Trade Organisation (WTO) makes the rules about 'free trade' in agriculture and means richer countries can control world prices and keep much of the profits for themselves. 'Free trade' for multi-national companies means global markets are opened up for their products. 'Free trade' rules for smaller farmers in the developing world and in Britain mean they struggle to make a profit.

Unless we buy fairly-traded goods, we are supporting the 'middle man' – the importer, the food processing company or the super-market supplier – not the farmer. Buying fairly-traded products, such as coffee, tea, cocoa, honey and bananas, puts money back into local communities to give everyone a better standard of life. Farmers are guaranteed a fair price for their products, enabling them to feed and educate their families.

Did you know?
Aren't GM crops the way to feed the world?

There are more than 800 million people in the world who don't have enough to eat. But according to aid agencies the problem is poverty, not food shortages. Intensive farming, GM or not, destroys soil fertility. Small-scale farmers need help to grow food in sustainable and less intensive ways, to maintain crop diversity and feed their families at low cost. This is the way to ensure everyone has enough to eat.

In Haiti, most coffee farmers are small-holders. Café Direct pays them more than twice the usual rate for their coffee. These fair trade prices have funded a school, a football pitch, a meeting room and several horses for one co-op on the island.

Your children's food

Children are more susceptible to toxic effects because their bodies are still growing. Because of this, pesticide residues in processed baby food are now banned. But residues remain in fruit and vegetables – and children should be eating these for their health. Buy organic food for your children when you can. Let your supermarket know you don't want pesticide residues in your food.

Organic versus local

Most of the organic food sold in supermarkets is imported, some from the other side of the world. It doesn't make sense to damage the environment by using large quantities of fuel to import organic food when we could grow it locally.

Write to your supermarket asking for policies to support local producers. In the meantime, find local alternatives if you can. Keep yourself informed about food issues and weigh up the arguments.

Friends of the Earth's Real Food Campaign

Here's how we are working towards a truly sustainable future.

Friends of the Earth has a vision for a new future for food and farming. We want to see a fair deal for farmers and consumers. We want the Government to act so that farmers are able to manage the countryside sustainably and provide high-quality food for a fair income.

Environment

We want investment in sustainable agriculture like organic farming, so that the environment is protected and wildlife in our countryside can flourish.

Rural communities

We want regeneration in rural communities, with more farming jobs in less-intensive production, better public transport in rural areas, more local food sold locally in farmers' markets or local shops, and a fair income for farmers who farm sustainably.

Food safety

Pesticide residues should be eliminated from our food. All GM ingredients in food and animal products should be labelled if they are detectable. No further GM trials or commercial planting should be allowed until laws to prevent contamination and place strict liability for all harm arising on the biotech companies are in force.

Organic targets

Friends of the Earth is calling for more support for local organic food initiatives, to make organic food more accessible to more people. Safe, nutritious, healthy food should be available to all.

Contact Friends of the Earth for more information about our Real Food Campaign and how to join us. Full campaign information, briefings and reports are on our website. Information Service Freephone: 0808 800 1111 Email: info@foe.co.uk or visit www.foe.co.uk/campaigns/real_food/

Friends of the Earth is:
- the UK's most influential national environmental campaigning organisation
- the most extensive environmental network in the world, with almost one million supporters across five continents and over 60 national organisations worldwide
- a unique network of campaigning local groups, working in over 200 communities throughout England, Wales and Northern Ireland
- dependent on individuals for over 90 per cent of its income. Friends of the Earth inspires solutions to environmental problems, which make life better for people

The hidden dangers in our food

By Isabel Oakeshott, *Evening Standard*

New research reveals the full dangers of additives in our food and drink. A study by the Consumers Association shows how unappetising additives in regular use include wood chip, chalk and pigment from dried insect bodies.

Consumer watchdogs claimed many food labels read 'more like a chemistry experiment than something you'd want to eat' and called for far clearer labelling.

Foods highlighted in the study include Golden Wonder crispy bacon Wheat Crunchies, which contain flavourings and colouring but no bacon; Rowntree's sugar-free strawberry flavour jelly, which contains no strawberries, and Calypso Freeze-pops, which contain a raft of flavourings, stabilisers, preservatives and sweeteners. Millions of shoppers try to avoid products with artificial flavourings and preservatives amid mounting health fears. One-third of the 2000 people surveyed by *Consumer Which?* magazine said they did not want these foods.

Additives have been linked to skin rashes, asthma attacks, headaches, behaviour problems and even brain tumours. But offenders – many of them foodstuffs targeted at children – contain them, often listed as E numbers and used as a substitute for 'real' ingredients. Amanda Bristow, who compiled the report, said: 'Food additives can be labelled with either their E number, or their chemical name, or both. It is no surprise that most people we asked could not identify all the additives on an ingredients list.'

Health groups reacted with dismay, warning that certain additives could trigger devastating allergies and illnesses.

Calls for clearer labels were backed by the British Dietetic Association. Dietitian Azmina Govinda said: 'Manufacturers should use more simple language so that people know what they are getting.'

Additives are used to preserve, add colour, flavour or texture to food and drink. However, campaigners say not enough is known about their side effects.

• This article first appeared in the *Evening Standard*, February 2004.

Food crimes

Information from the Co-op

The seven food crimes

The impetus to cut costs, produce and sell more underpins the way the world rears its animals, grows its crops and manufactures and markets its food, sometimes with alarming effects. Indeed, these perceived food-related felonies are usually committed with the full force of the law and the scientific community working against consumers' views. The trouble is they just don't recognise that science and the law frequently lag behind consumer opinion, which often condemns as abhorrent the practices the Co-op has identified as the 'seven food crimes' . . .

1. Blackmail – The insidious targeting of the public by global big business putting huge marketing muscle behind products that fail to fit in with healthy eating advice.

Parents, in particular, feel they are in competition with advertisers who they believe deliberately target their children. Advertising and promotion fan the flames of 'pester power'. The Co-op found that 73 per cent of children ask their parents to buy sweets and crisps they have seen advertised, and only 19 per cent of children give up when their parents say no. Meanwhile 71 per cent of kids have bought something on the strength of a free gift or special offer.

2. Contamination – The unnecessary use of chemicals on land and in livestock – interference with nature's way.

Consumers have no faith in the premise that chemicals improve quality. Just one quarter of people believe pesticides deliver better quality fruit and vegetables. This uneasiness is exacerbated by the fact that shoppers feel powerless to avoid them – 64 per cent believe washing food will not remove pesticides. Feeding animals with growth-promoting antibiotics met with the disapproval of 87 per cent of consumers in the Co-op survey.

3. GBH* – The disregard of animal rights to keep costs down or, even worse, to pamper our taste buds with so called 'luxuries'.

Intensive farming of livestock has transformed the lives of farm animals. The desire to increase yield has been placed above all else with the result that for poultry, females could be crammed into cages, males could be gassed at birth. Some animals literally never see the light of day until they are sent for slaughter. Geese are force-fed to produce foie gras. 84 per cent are concerned that animals are not treated properly. But the public's disquiet goes beyond passive pity. In total, 61 per cent 'want to know more' about the conditions animals are kept in, although nearly a fifth prefer ignorance because they feel powerless to change the situation.

*Grievous Bodily Harm

4. Vandalism – The destruction of the planet by the intensification of food production systems.

Consumers seem worried that the ecosystem is being irreversibly damaged by the profit motive of the food industry with potentially catastrophic results. The survey found 72 per cent believe the environment is being damaged by global food production. 70 per cent of consumers disapprove of the application of human sewage on farmland as a fertiliser and 82 per cent of people are concerned that wildlife suffers as a result of intensive farming. What's more, consumers are unimpressed by the supposed gains made by such methods – 74 per cent feel too much attention is paid to what fruit and vegetables look like. And on the heated issue of GM, 91 per cent disapproved of products made with this technology.

5. Cannibalism – The practice of permitting animals to be fed with the remains of their own species, or herbivores with animal by-products, or giving animals feed made from the blood of other animals.

Despite the revulsion to these practices expressed by consumers, Government officials admitted as recently as April 2000 that for certain species this is still allowed. Consumers seem well aware of such abuses. Co-op research found 55 per cent, for example, familiar with the practice of making feed from animal blood. Needless to say, they do not approve. 86 per cent disapprove of

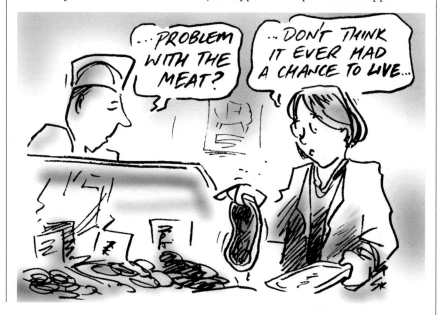

...PROBLEM WITH THE MEAT?

...DON'T THINK IT EVER HAD A CHANCE TO LIVE...

animal blood and 90 per cent disapprove of the use of chicken feathers. Predictably, 73 per cent of consumers believe these practices have a 'bad effect' on what we eat. And when asked whether BSE was just an isolated health scare, 83 per cent of consumers disagree and suggest 'there are others'.

6. Pillage – The careless exploitation of countries, cultures and creeds by multinational concerns milking the so-called global economy.

Whilst welcoming year-round availability, people seem concerned that the laissez-faire development of the global economy is destroying livelihoods, communities and the environment. 85 per cent of people feel big multinational companies have too much power over what we eat. 89 per cent think that multinationals do not act in the interests of the general public, 81 per cent think that it is wrong for third world farmers to be exploited to bring us cheap food and 64 per cent worry that the standards of farming will not be as strict as they are in Britain.

7. Fraud – The deliberate assault on the taste and appearance of our food.

The Co-op survey found that 74 per cent think artificial colours are unnecessary or even harmful and 93 per cent believe people have the right to know everything that has happened to their food, not just about the ingredients on the label. 82 per cent of consumers feel additives and flavourings used in convenience food often hide the taste of natural ingredients.

Too much to swallow?
Consumers give their views
How do consumers feel about these food crimes? Are they well informed? Do they feel powerless to change anything? Do they care? If so, whom do they blame? The Co-op asked them for their views.

The benefits
Modern food methods are not without their dividends. Few dispute that. The question is how we balance these advantages against the ethical and environmental costs involved. Consumers overwhelmingly welcome the choice, cost, convenience and quantity of goods available.

But it's a minority who are unquestioning about the effects of commercialisation.

'I think it's wonderful, I really do. I love eating what I want when I want.'

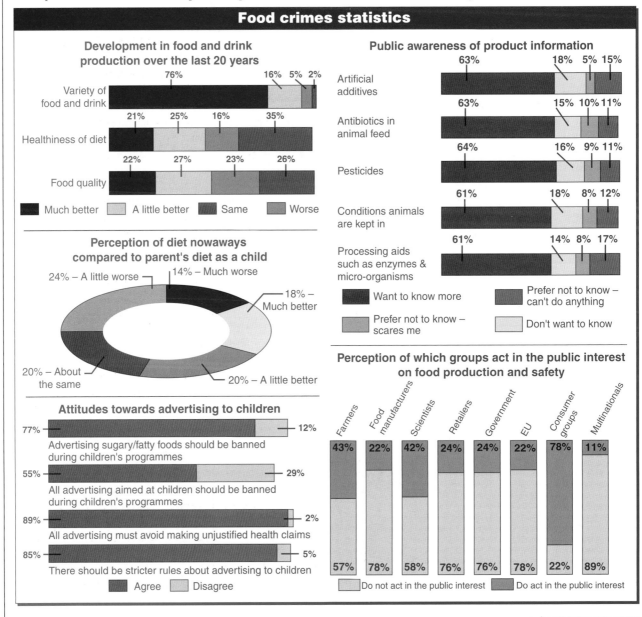

Food crimes statistics

Development in food and drink production over the last 20 years

- Variety of food and drink: Much better 76%, A little better 16%, Same 5%, Worse 2%
- Healthiness of diet: Much better 21%, A little better 25%, Same 16%, Worse 35%
- Food quality: Much better 22%, A little better 27%, Same 23%, Worse 26%

Legend: Much better | A little better | Same | Worse

Perception of diet nowaways compared to parent's diet as a child

- 14% – Much worse
- 18% – Much better
- 20% – A little better
- 24% – A little worse
- 20% – About the same

Attitudes towards advertising to children

- Advertising sugary/fatty foods should be banned during children's programmes: Agree 77%, Disagree 12%
- All advertising aimed at children should be banned during children's programmes: Agree 55%, Disagree 29%
- All advertising must avoid making unjustified health claims: Agree 89%, Disagree 2%
- There should be stricter rules about advertising to children: Agree 85%, Disagree 5%

Legend: Agree | Disagree

Public awareness of product information

- Artificial additives: 63% | 18% | 5% | 15%
- Antibiotics in animal feed: 63% | 15% | 10% | 11%
- Pesticides: 64% | 16% | 9% | 11%
- Conditions animals are kept in: 61% | 18% | 8% | 12%
- Processing aids such as enzymes & micro-organisms: 61% | 14% | 8% | 17%

Legend: Want to know more | Prefer not to know – scares me | Prefer not to know – can't do anything | Don't want to know

Perception of which groups act in the public interest on food production and safety

	Farmers	Food manufacturers	Scientists	Retailers	Government	EU	Consumer groups	Multinationals
Do act in the public interest	43%	22%	42%	24%	24%	22%	78%	11%
Do not act in the public interest	57%	78%	58%	76%	76%	78%	22%	89%

'We can't go back to the days when mum was at home all day cooking three meals a day.'

Information

Overall consumers feel frustrated by their lack of knowledge of what goes into their food and how it is made. Although some express an 'ignorance is bliss' attitude which permits them to enjoy their meals without guilt, others prefer not to know because they feel powerless to effect change or because it 'scares' them. However, the majority prefer to be able to make informed choices.

'I deliberately ignore some of it as I want to eat meat and I find it too disturbing to watch. If I watched enough of those programmes, I'd probably go vegetarian.'

'They are too frightened to tell us what is in the food. No one in their right mind would eat a chicken which has been pumped full of antibiotics.'

The culprits

It appears the public have lost confidence in most groups associated with the food industry. They believe the profit motive generally scores over the public interest. Multinationals rate especially poorly, with retailers, manufacturers and the government faring little better. However, the public do not absolve themselves from blame. Some believe their own apathy adds to the malaise.

'(For the supermarkets) produce has got to be a certain size, shape and colour … so if the product isn't up to scratch then the farmer just has to destroy a lot of it.'

'Battery chickens, battery cows … everything is intensively kept. Piglets are taken away a couple of hours old … sows are constantly having piglets … to me that is intensive farming. It's a big problem.'

'I was shocked when I found out it was already in American soya. That sort of hit me. I thought – how could they have done this without asking me or telling me first.'

'I saw a documentary on how they were kept. I'm not an animal lover but it made me cry. It was evil. They can't

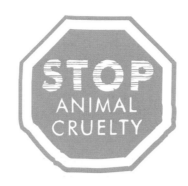

even stand up properly. They can't stretch their wings.'

The perpetrators

The advertising industry argues that parents should control what their children eat, yet a welling anger and sense of powerlessness comes through in parents' attitudes to the targeting of children by the food industry. Parents are split about whether children's diets are better than in years gone by, but, according to a 1999 report in *Public Health and Nutrition* (the Nutrition Society's publication), 40 years ago children ate substantially more bread and vegetables and less sugar and soft drinks, so their diets were arguably better for them than what children eat today. However, parents are under pressure to buy 'junk' foods. Pester power is fuelled by the marketing of big corporations and it's parents who bear the brunt. When Sweden takes over the EU Presidency it is expected to press for its own ban on advertising to children to be extended to the rest of Europe – a move which the UK advertising industry is expected to oppose.

'If you have a two-year-old lying on the ground and a five-year-old screaming, I give in, I just want to get out of the shop.'

'If we don't get it for them then we are bad, we are cruel, we are the misers.'

'I don't want them to hassle me in the supermarket… I want my children to grow up sensibly and not be led by advertisers.'

The fightback

Consumers often feel powerless and want to know more when it comes to food crimes. Yet they are crying out for the means to act. Small individual acts of defiance are made every time a shopper boycotts a certain product or opts for an alternative such as free-range eggs. The most successful example is the consumer backlash against GM. But price still holds them back and the overall impression is that the public would respond to a lead from those within the food industry.

Active purchasing of certain products

31% Organic products
29% Free-range meat
24% Meat from animals reared on natural diet
22% Better quality convenience foods
62% Free-range eggs
20% Fair-trade products
27% None

Barriers to purchasing these products

46% Can't afford them
13% Not worth the money
6% Don't know where to buy them
9% Can't find them locally
2% Look less appetising
6% Taste is no different
1% Taste is worse

'I dig my head in the sand because the issues are so huge. But if I felt they were going to do something about it I would be delighted and I would shop there more.'

'If everybody stopped buying GM foods then they wouldn't bother. It wouldn't be viable financially for them to do it.'

■ The Co-op commissioned market research by NOPConsumer who interviewed 1,216 adults (523 of whom were parents) and 293 children under 11 years old. Group discussions were also conducted by Wardle McLean Strategic Research Consultancy with adults (including parents) and children under 11 years old. The research was conducted in February and March 2000.

■ The above information is an extract from *Food Crimes, A consumer perspective on the ethics of modern food production* produced by the CO-OP.
© CWS Ltd

Remote control

Who polices the chemicals added to our food, and who makes the rules? Sally Kinnes finds out

Every week, between 100 and 250 packages arrive, usually by courier, at Hampshire Scientific Services in Portsmouth. Sent by officers from trading standards, environmental health, port authorities and the like, they contain samples of food and drink, bagged and tagged like police evidence. One of these recently contained samples of chicken tikka masala. Their arrival was the trigger for a tabloid scandal.

In the laboratory, the samples of Britain's favourite Indian dish were put on a glass plate, soaked in a solvent to separate the colours and, with state-of-the-art, high-performance liquid chromatography, the amount of colour was measured. Compared with levels permitted by the Colours in Food Regulations 1995, they were way off the scale – 58 out of 102 chicken tikka masala samples tested on this occasion had 'illegal and potentially dangerous' levels of colourants. 'It's quite frightening,' says Rachel New, a scientific consultant who helped perform the analysis. 'Surveys like this have been carried out before, and the worrying thing is, it's not going away.'

This was the so-called 'Surrey Curry', sent by trading standards officers from Surrey county council, who had visited restaurants throughout the county. Like environmental health officers, who check the environment in which food is produced, trading standards officers enforce the law. A team a few thousand strong, they are the food police. They swoop on meals-on-wheels and school canteens, supermarkets and corner shops, to ensure food complies with the law. Slipping in unannounced and anonymous, they take informal samples for testing and if they find, for example, a suspect sausage, they get the manufacturer's or retailer's permission to take a formal sample, which could be used in court. The sausage is then split into three. One piece is retained for

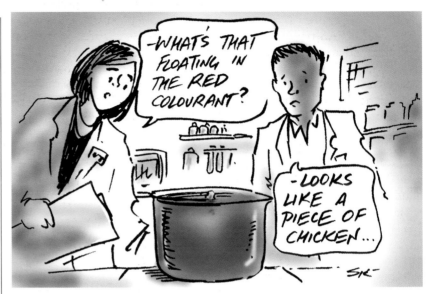

testing by the retailer or manufacturer. One is sent to the public analyst, a scientist at a lab such as Hampshire Scientific Services. The third piece – the so-called 'referee sample' – is kept by trading standards and, in the event of a disputed test result, this bit of the banger goes to have its ingredients scrutinised by the Laboratory of the Government Chemist (LGC) in Teddington. Depending on what is found, trading standards may prosecute, caution or advise.

Like environmental health officers, who check the environment in which food is produced, trading standards officers enforce the law. A team a few thousand strong, they are the food police

---

Other parts of the food supply chain are subject to other types of policing. Four times a year, the pesticide residues committee, chaired by Dr Ian Brown, carries out a survey to see how much of the pesticides farmers spray on crops remains in fruit and vegetables and prepared food. The Meat Hygiene Service tests for residues in meat from slaughterhouses, and the State Veterinary Service (SVS) inspects veterinary medicine records, on farms and in vets' surgeries.

Taken all together, these are the foot soldiers in the war against illegal food. If your local Chinese takeaway is illegally overdoing the monosodium glutamate, if your apples have too many chemical residues, or your chicken tikka masala is much redder than it ought to be, these are the people we rely on to find out, and put a stop to it.

It is an enormous job and there are several constraints on their work. Unsurprisingly, one problem is money. 'Their budgets are squeezed all the time,' says Tim Lang, professor of food policy at City University in London. 'That's been a long-running concern for me.'

According to Julie Barrett, a director of the Chartered Institute of Environmental Health (CIEH), the problem is exacerbated by a target-oriented testing regime. 'Local authorities used to decide their own inspections, but now targets are imposed by the Food Standards Agency. That means resources are deflected from other things, like food hygiene training.'

Then there is the problem of penalties. 'Illegal meat is a huge problem, but there are not sufficient penalties to act as a deterrent,' Barrett says. 'We have to prosecute under Conspiracy to Defraud, which was never intended to be used for food.' The CIEH is also lobbying for food premises to be licensed before they can be opened. 'Anyone can open a restaurant, and it could be the most squalid, horrible hole, but until someone from environmental health stumbles across it, it will not be inspected.'

Enforcing the enforcers are the staff of the Food and Veterinary Office. If trading standards do the equivalent of walking the beat and pulling up offenders, these are the chief inspectors, ensuring they do their job. The majority of food legislation is made at EU level and it is up to the Dublin-based Food and Veterinary Office to send inspectors to ensure all member states are enforcing the rules.

So who makes up the rules? Ultimately, what's allowed in our food is judged by an army of scientific committees, reporting to the Food Standards Agency (FSA), the food safety watchdog in the UK, and to the newly formed European Food Safety Authority. Set up by the European Parliament and Council Regulation (EC) No178/2002 in January 2002, following a series of food scares, the EFSA will eventually move from its temporary Brussels base to Parma in Italy. Its task is to provide independent scientific advice on food safety issues. So, for example, its scientific panel on food additives, flavourings, processing aids and materials in contact with food makes a risk assessment of a specific chemical and provides the European parliament with the scientific base for legislation. But chemicals tend to be assessed on an individual basis. 'Individual committees look at individual chemicals, and as a consumer, it's very difficult to get a full picture of how they accumulate together,' says Sue Davies, the Consumers' Association's principal policy adviser on food. 'It's something we'd like to see the FSA get better at.'

As for the legislation itself, it's an alphabet soup of acts, European directives and regulations and amendments. The main piece of UK legislation is the Food Safety Act, but according to Brown at the pesticide residues committee, pesticides come under Pesticides Regulation 1986 (as amended), part of the Agriculture Act. And just to deal with the complexity of additives in food, there are three pieces of legislation: the Sweeteners in Food Regulations 1995 (as amended), the Colours in Food Regulations 1995 (as amended) and the Miscellaneous Food Additives Regulations 1995 (as amended).

Ultimately, what's allowed in our food is judged by an army of scientific committees, reporting to the Food Standards Agency (FSA), the food safety watchdog in the UK

Additives are divided into six groups: antioxidants (synthetic antioxidants can be added to foods that contain fats to stop them going off); colours; emulsifiers, stabilisers, gelling agents and thickeners; flavourings; preservatives; and sweeteners. Every additive that is legally permitted has an E number, the E indicating that it has been approved for use in Europe. With 45 colours, 12 flavours and 15 anti-oxidants permitted in food, some products are made of little else. According to a Consumers' Association report last year, if you extract the additives from things like Tizer or Calypso, water and sugar is all that is left.

There is, then, a complicated network of controls, spread from Ireland to Italy, designed to decide what level of chemicals should legally be allowed in food, and to catch those who exceed them. The arrival of the Food Standards Agency – something for which the Consumers' Association campaigned hard – has made responsibilities clearer, Davies says, but the association is waiting to see if its new European sister is as open with its decision-making as is promised.

Lang at City University says the real issue isn't about controls, though. 'It's about the need for more independent food scientists. In the mid-19th century, modern food chemistry began by acting on people's behalf. What we've got now is chemistry that, by and large, works for the food industry. People in mainstream public health say the problem is not adulterated food, it's heart disease, cancer and diabetes, and they are absolutely right. But the point people like me have been making for years is that the modern legalised adulteration and legalised contamination of food is what enables foods full of hidden fats and sugars to be sold looking like real food. That is the flipside of the coin.'

■ This article first appeared in *The Guardian*, 15 May 2004.

© Sally Kinnes

On-the-spot inspections

Number and type of inspections carried out and infringments established (in accordance with Article 14 of Directive 89/397/EEC) in 2000

Number of establishments	603,328
Number of establishments inspected	385,507
Number of inspections	544,840
Number of establishments committing infringements*	174,417
Hygiene general (handling procedures, equipment and condition of premises	302
Hygiene of personnel (in conformity with article 8 of the Control Directive)	12
Composition (including raw material and additives)	107
Contamination (other than microbiological)	61
Labelling and presentation	224
Others	47

* Only the ones which have led to formal action by the competent authorities.

Source: Food Standards Agency

KEY FACTS

- Healthy eating and a healthful way of life are important to how we look, feel and how much we enjoy life. (p. 1)

- The latest figures, based on official data from the Health Survey for England for 2001/2, show that more than one in four children are overweight and 6-7% are classified as obese. (p. 3)

- Few teenagers associate eating with regular meal times and most lack the skill to prepare anything more than a ready meal. (p. 4)

- 8 guidelines for a healthy diet:
  - Enjoy your food
  - Eat a variety of different foods
  - Eat the right amount to be a healthy weight
  - Eat plenty of foods rich in starch and fibre
  - Eat plenty of fruit and vegetables
  - Don't eat too many foods that contain a lot of fat
  - Don't have sugary foods and drinks too often
  - If you drink alcohol, drink sensibly (p. 5)

- Eat breakfast and don't skip meals. You'll be more alert and your metabolism will be better. People who eat breakfast regularly are more likely to be slim than people who skip it. (p. 8)

- Obesity now affects 21 per cent of men and 23 per cent of women in the UK. A further 46 per cent of men and 33 per cent of women are overweight. (p. 9)

- More than half the world's population fails to do 30 minutes of moderate activity a day. (p. 11)

- Whenever we eat more than our body needs, we put on weight. This is because our body stores the energy we don't use up, usually as fat. (p. 12)

- Breakfast is one of the easiest meals in which to get calcium into the diet through the consumption of milk and dairy products such as yogurt. A serving of milk on cereal can provide up to half our daily calcium requirement. (p. 15)

- The average salt intake is currently 9.5g a day (about 2 teaspoons), we should be having much less than this – the recommended intake is just 6g a day. (p. 16)

- There is overwhelming evidence of the health benefits of eating fruit and vegetables, particularly in reducing the risks of heart disease, and some cancers. (p. 17)

- 'Children are bombarded with messages that promote food high in fat, salt and sugar. The evidence shows that these messages do influence children. Eating too much of these foods is storing up health problems for their future. (p. 19)

- Food labelling is strictly governed by law. A food can't claim to be 'reduced calorie' unless it is much lower in calories than the usual version. (p. 23)

- The battle for better labelling is not new. But the Consumers' Association (CA), which has been campaigning for honest information for several years, believes labels matter more now than ever before. (p. 24)

- Each year it is estimated that as many as 5.5 million people in the UK may suffer from food-borne illnesses – that's 1 in 10 people. (p. 27)

- In 1939 there were half a million farms in the UK employing 15 per cent of the population. In 2000 only two per cent of the population still worked in agriculture. (p. 31)

- 18,000 jobs in agriculture were lost in 2002 and many small farms went out of business. Some 65,000 people left farming in the six years up to 2002. (p. 32)

- Most of the organic food sold in supermarkets is imported, some from the other side of the world. It doesn't make sense to damage the environment by using large quantities of fuel to import organic food when we could grow it locally. (p. 33)

- Consumer watchdogs claim many food labels read 'more like a chemistry experiment than something you'd want to eat' and called for far clearer labelling. (p. 34)

- Consumers seem worried that the ecosystem is being irreversibly damaged by the profit motive of the food industry with potentially catastrophic results. The survey found 72 per cent believe the environment is being damaged by global food production. (p. 35)

- The advertising industry argues that parents should control what their children eat, yet a welling anger and sense of powerlessness comes through in parents' attitudes to the targeting of children by the food industry. (p. 37)

- Like environmental health officers, who check the environment in which food is produced, trading standards officers enforce the law. A team a few thousand strong, they are the food police. (p. 38)

- Ultimately, what's allowed in our food is judged by an army of scientific committees, reporting to the Food Standards Agency (FSA), the food safety watchdog in the UK. (p. 39)

ADDITIONAL RESOURCES

You might like to contact the following organisations for further information. Due to the increasing cost of postage, many organisations cannot respond to enquiries unless they receive a stamped, addressed envelope.

British Nutrition Foundation (BNF)
High Holborn House
52-54 High Holborn
London, WC1V 6RQ
Tel: 020 7404 6504
Fax: 020 7404 6747
E-mail: postbox@nutrition.org.uk
Website: www.nutrition.org.uk
The BNF is an independent charity which provides reliable information and advice on nutrition and related health matters.

Co-operative Group (CWS) Limited
New Century House
Manchester, M60 4ES
Tel: 0161 834 1212
Website: www.co-op.co.uk

Dietetic Association
5th Floor, Charles House
148/9 Great Charles Street,
Queensway
Birmingham, B3 3HT
Tel: 0121 200 8080
Fax: 0121 200 8081
E-mail: info@bda.uk.com
Website: www.bda.uk.com
The British Dietetic Association, established in 1936, was formed to provide training and facilities for State Registered Dietitians.

European Food Information Council (EUFIC)
1 Place des Pyramides 75001
Paris, France
Tel: + 33 140 20 44 40
Fax: + 33 140 20 44 41
E-mail: eufic@eufic.org
Website: www.eufic.org
EUFIC has been established to provide science-based information on foods and food-related topics i.e. nutrition and health, food safety and quality and biotechnology in food for the attention of European consumers.

Food and Drink Federation
6 Catherine Street
London, WC2B 5JJ
Tel: 020 7836 2460
Fax: 020 7836 0580
Website: www.fdf.org.uk
Produces publications and surveys on food and biotechnology.

The Food Commission
94 White Lion Street
London, N1 9PF
Tel: 020 7837 2250
Fax: 020 7837 1141
E-mail:
enquiries@foodcomm.org.uk
Website: www.foodcomm.org.uk
The Food Commission is committed to ensuring good quality food for all.

Food Standards Agency
Aviation House
125 Kingsway
London, WC2B 6NH.
Tel: 020 7276 8000
Website: www.food.gov.uk
The Agency was been created to: 'protect public health from risks which may arise in connection with the consumption of food, and otherwise to protect the interests of consumers in relation to food'.

Friends of the Earth (FOE)
26-28 Underwood Street
London, N1 7JQ
Tel: 020 7490 1555
Fax: 020 7490 0881
E-mail: info@foe.co.uk
Website: www.foe.co.uk
Friends of the Earth publishes a comprehensive range of leaflets, books, briefings and reports.

Health Development Agency
Holborn Gate
330 High Holborn
London, WC1V 7BA
Tel: 020 7430 0850
Fax: 020 7413 8900
Website: www.hda.nhs.uk
The HDA identifies the evidence of what works to improve people's health and reduce health inequalities.

International Obesity TaskForce (IOTF)
231 North Gower Street
London, NW1 2NS
Tel: 020 7691 1900
Fax: 020 7387 6033
E-mail: obesity@iotf.org
Website: www.iotf.org
www.iaso.org
The IOTF is working to alert the world of the growing health crisis threatened by soaring levels of obesity.

The Soil Association
Bristol House
40-56 Victoria Street
Bristol, BS1 6BY
Tel: 0117 929 0661
Fax; 0117 925 2504
E-mail: info@soilassociation.org
Website: www.soilassociation.org
Works to educate the general public about organic agriculture, gardening and food, and their benefits for both human health and the environment.

Sustain
94 White Lion Street
London, N1 9PF
Tel: 020 7837 1228
Fax: 020 7837 1141
E-mail: sustain@sustainweb.org
Website: www.sustainweb.org
Sustain policies and practices that enhance the health and welfare of people and animal, improve the working and living environment, enrich society and culture and promote equity.

YouthNet UK
2-3 Upper Street
Islington
London, N1 0PH
Tel: 020 7226 8008
Fax: 020 7226 8118
E-mail: info@thesite.org
Website: www.thesite.org
TheSite.org is produced and managed by YouthNet UK. TheSite.org aims to offer the best guide to life for young adults, aged 16-25.

INDEX

ACKNOWLEDGEMENTS

The publisher is grateful for permission to reproduce the following material.

While every care has been taken to trace and acknowledge copyright, the publisher tenders its apology for any accidental infringement or where copyright has proved untraceable. The publisher would be pleased to come to a suitable arrangement in any such case with the rightful owner.

Chapter One: Healthy Eating

Adult nutrition, © EUFIC, *UK child obesity crisis*, © International Obesity TaskForce (IOTF), *Overweight children*, © International Obesity TaskForce (IOTF), *Teenagers 'too idle' to bother with good food*, © Telegraph Group Limited, London 2004, *Consumption of fruit and vegetables*, © Crown copyright is reproduced with the permission of Her Majesty's Stationery Office, *Healthy eating*, © British Nutrition Foundation (BNF), *A balanced diet*, © TheSite.org, *Junk food timebomb*, © *The Observer*, *Food and drinks consumed*, © Crown copyright is reproduced with the permission of Her Majesty's Stationery Office, *New food bill to combat child obesity*, © 2004 Associated Newspapers Ltd, *How to be a healthy weight*, © Food Standards Agency, *Food quality and your health*, © Soil Association, *Organic crops*, © Crown copyright is reproduced with the permission of Her Majesty's Stationery Office, *Is breakfast important?*, © British Nutrition Foundation (BNF), *Salt and health*, © The British Dietetic Association, *Salt use*, © Crown copyright is reproduced with the permission of Her Majesty's Stationery Office, *What is so good about fruit and vegetables?*, © Sustain, *Four nutrition myths*, © EUFIC, *Food promotion to children*, © Crown copyright is reproduced with the permission of Her Majesty's Stationery Office, *Parent power works!*, © The Food Commission.

Chapter Two: Food Safety

Understanding the food label, © The British Dietetic Association, *What do labels tell me?*, © Crown copyright is reproduced with the permission of Her Majesty's Stationery Office, *Reading between the lines*, © Health Development Agency, *Consumer attitudes towards food*, © Crown copyright is reproduced with the permission of Her Majesty's Stationery Office, *Food poisoning*, © Food and Drink Federation, *Food poisoning statistics*, © Food and Drink Federation, *Healthy eating branded 'illegal'*, © 2004 Associated Newspapers Ltd, *Food and farming*, © Friends of the Earth, *The hidden dangers in our food*, © 2004 Associated Newspapers Ltd, *Food crimes*, © CWS Ltd, *Food crimes statistics*, © CWS Ltd, *Remote control*, © Sally Kinnes, *On-the-spot inspections*, © Food Standards Agency.

Photographs and illustrations:

Pages 1, 17, 27, 35, 38: Simon Kneebone; pages 6, 18, 24; Angelo Madrid; pages 8, 21, 32: Pumpkin House; pages 13, 23, 30: Don Hatcher; pages 15, 22: Bev Aisbett.

Craig Donnellan
Cambridge
September, 2004